BEHÇET'S DISEASE

LICENSE, DISCLAIMER OF LIABILITY, AND LIMITED WARRANTY

BEHÇET'S DISEASE

Joanne Zeis

MERCURY LEARNING AND INFORMATION
Dulles, Virginia
Boston, Massachusetts
New Delhi

Publisher: David Pallai
MERCURY LEARNING AND INFORMATION
22841 Quicksilver Drive
Dulles, VA 20166
info@merclearning.com
www.merclearning.com
1-800-758-3756

This book is printed on acid-free paper.

Joanne Zeis. *Behçet's Disease.*
ISBN: 978-1-938549-40-3

Library of Congress Control Number: 2014950129
171819654

Printed in the United States of America

Our titles are available for adoption, license, or bulk purchase by
associations, universities, corporations, etc. Digital versions of this title may
be purchased at www.authorcloudware.com or other e-vendors.
For additional information or companion e-files, please contact the Customer
Service Dept. at 1-800-232-0223 (toll free) or info@merclearning.com.

Contents

Foreword

When patients are first suspected to have an illness, or when they receive a diagnosis—particularly one they have never heard of—a number of questions quickly come to mind. Writing these questions down for a discussion with the provider is always a good idea, but all questions may not be answered, and other concerns will come up after the visit. No longer are those at risk satisfied with, "Don't worry, things will be all right," despite confidence in or reputation of the provider. Meeting the needs of the patient means providing knowledge and understanding, along with appropriate reassurance of uncertainty or concern. Empowerment to participate in one's own health decisions is the foundation of patient-centered care.

For Behçet's disease, a partnership between trusted physician and patient works best to ensure the best patient outcomes and patient experience. The two-way sharing of information will lead to critical teamwork and a greater fund of knowledge; it will also result in a greater understanding of the interaction between the disorder and the individual. For Behçet's, as variable as it may be, this understanding is key to appropriate treatment.

Behçet's Disease answers 92 questions that those affected with this disorder would likely have, and it clarifies the disorder in 15 chapters. Disease variability and differences in risk between genders, ages, and populations is appropriately highlighted. The author updates and builds on an earlier work, *Essential Guide to Behçet's Disease* (2003). This new effort is available in e-format and print versions, and it takes advantage of links to online resources that greatly expand the available information, should the reader wish to explore questions further. What is unchanged is the author's passion as a Behçet's patient, researcher and advocate, to empower the reader with understanding and tools to meet and contain the challenges of this disease.

Kenneth T. Calamia, MD
Professor of Medicine
Mayo Clinic College of Medicine

Preface

It's ironic that my latest book about Behçet's is a compilation of frequently asked questions, because the question I'm asked **most** often is when I'm going to release a second edition of the *Essential Guide to Behçet's Disease*. While this new book isn't a second edition, it's an excellent supplement to the *Essential Guide's* wealth of information. It provides updates on treatments, pregnancy, Behçet's in the United States and Western Europe, guidelines to manage neuro-Behçet's, and over 85 more topics. It also tackles several new issues, like what happens when BD patients get tattoos.

This publication will be most helpful for people with Behçet's, healthcare providers facing their first Behçet's patient(s), and the caregivers and loved ones of people with BD. It's easy to tell a person with Behçet's that "it's all in your head," and walk away. However, it's always much kinder and gentler to say, "I don't understand what's happening, but let's learn about it together." This book is a great start.

Be well,
Joanne Zeis
October, 2014

Acknowledgments

This book would never have been possible without the support of the following people and groups:

Mike, Ben, and Sarah; the Executive Board of the American Behçet's Disease Association; Kenneth Calamia, MD, Mirta Avila Santos, MD, and Delfin Santos, MD, who reviewed the manuscript in advance; Lisa Jensen, MPH, for her painstaking and thorough edits; and C. Stephen Foster, MD, founder of Massachusetts Eye Research and Surgery Institution, for his longstanding support of my work and for providing the elusive diagnosis that started my journey.

I'm grateful to David Pallai and Mercury Learning for the chance to publish this book as part of the *MyModernHealth FAQs* series. By guaranteeing worldwide distribution, it puts much-needed information into the hands of people who might not otherwise have access to it.

For Behçet's patients and support groups in the United States and around the world, your emails and posts are the first thing I read in the morning and the last information I see at the end of the day. We're all in this together.

An overview of Behçet's disease

1. What is Behçet's disease?

Behçet's disease (BD) is a rare, chronic autoimmune illness. In the United States, a rare disease is one that affects fewer than 200,000 people. Approximately 15,000–20,000 Americans have been diagnosed with Behçet's.

Behçet's is not contagious, so you can't catch it from someone else. It usually starts during a person's 20s and 30s, but it can affect people of any age, from newborn babies to the elderly. Behçet's causes vasculitis, which is the inflammation of blood vessels. Wherever this inflammation occurs in the body is where a person may have symptoms.

Researchers believe people with Behçet's have a *genetic predisposition* for the disease, but some type of trigger is needed to set it off—like something in the environment, or some type of virus or bacteria—before the person starts having symptoms. This genetic predisposition is a higher chance, but not a guarantee, of developing the disease. It's based on the genes you've received from both sides of your family.

Some experts think of Behçet's as *autoinflammatory* rather than autoimmune. Read about the difference between autoimmune and autoinflammatory diseases at http://www.niams.nih.gov/HEALTH_INFO/Autoinflammatory/default.asp

Researchers think streptococcal viruses may be involved as triggers, but it hasn't been proven. Heat shock proteins (HSP) and various bacteria have also been suggested.

Behçet's has a classic group of three symptoms: oral *aphthous* (app-thus) ulcers, genital aphthous ulcers and *uveitis* (you-vee-EYE-tis, a type of eye inflammation). As we'll see in this book, though, there is a wider range of symptoms than the top three mentioned here.

The Turkish dermatologist, Hulusi Behçet, often gets credit for publishing the first accounts of the illness in 1937, although Benediktos Adamantiades (a Greek ophthalmologist) wrote about a patient with these symptoms in 1931. Even Hippocrates noticed Behçet's-like symptoms in a case in the fifth century BC.

People with Behçet's disease have symptom flare-ups that come and go in cycles. Some of these flare-ups may be mild, but some can be severe and painful. Patients may be symptom-free for weeks or months, but then have their lives interrupted by flares that last for days, weeks, or much longer. This is the same type of pattern that happens to people with diseases like lupus or MS.

With time, many BD patients start to notice the triggers that set off their flares. Flares caused by strong emotional stress, menstrual periods and too much physical activity are common. Some people are affected by certain foods, or by high heat and humidity or other weather patterns, but very little research has been done on these topics. Pay attention to the timing of your own symptoms by keeping a health record or journal; both you and your doctor may find it helpful. Take pictures of any skin or mouth lesions to show your doctor in case these symptoms go away before your next appointment.

Most people with Behçet's have symptoms for their whole lives. Serious health issues, if they happen, may mean going into the hospital; however, research shows some patients may have *fewer* BD-related health problems as they get older. They may even go into remission,[2] where their symptoms stop. Unfortunately, it's hard to predict which way any individual case will go.

How is "Behçet's" pronounced? The correct Turkish pronunciation is Beh CHETS, although some researchers call it Beh CHET (without the "s"). Patients and English-speaking physicians often say Beh SHETS or *Bay* SHETS instead.

2. Is it Behçet's *disease* or Behçet's *syndrome*?

There is a long-standing argument among researchers about whether Behçet's is a disease or a syndrome (a group of signs and symptoms that often go together). Experts usually accept either term, but five times as many Behçet's-related articles in medical journals use "Behçet's disease" in their titles instead of "Behçet's syndrome."

Behçet's is also known by several other names: Adamantiades–Behçet's disease, triple-symptom complex, Morbus Behçet, and Silk Road disease, to name a few.

3. What kinds of doctors treat Behçet's?

Behçet's disease is a rheumatic illness: it causes inflammation and pain in different parts of the body, including the musculoskeletal system (made up of joints, bones, tendons, and muscles). That's why it's best for a rheumatologist to be the main medical contact for most Behçet's patients. You may also need to meet with one or more of the following specialists at some point, depending on your symptoms or complications: an ophthalmologist (eyes), dermatologist (skin), gastroenterologist (mostly the stomach/intestines), cardiologist (heart), neurologist (nervous system and brain), or immunologist (the immune system).

4. How can I find a doctor in my state or country who's familiar with treating Behçet's?

It's not always easy. Behçet's patient associations (such as the ABDA—the American Behçet's Disease Association) sometimes have listings of specialists recommended by other patients. Formal Behçet's patient groups are in the United Kingdom, China, France, Germany, Italy, Japan, Korea, Portugal, Spain, and Turkey. You can find informal Behçet's support groups on Facebook and other social networks. Once you join an online group, ask other members for the names of good doctors in your area. Since Behçet's isn't common in a lot of countries, it's rare for patients to have face-to-face meetings outside of medical conferences or fundraisers.

A dedicated Behçet's treatment center is helpful for people who need diagnosis and treatment. For example, the Behçet's Syndrome Center at the NYU Hospital for Joint Diseases in New York City has on-staff specialists and researchers committed to diagnosing, understanding and treating people with Behçet's in the United States. In the United Kingdom, there are three Behçet's Syndrome Centres of Excellence: Birmingham, Liverpool and London. Some other Behçet's specialty clinics can be found in Istanbul and Ankara (Turkey), Tehran (Iran)[1], and other countries.

Because Behçet's is a type of vasculitis, you may want to try a vasculitis center for diagnosis or treatment. The Vasculitis Foundation provides information and support for people with Behçet's and 16 other vascular diseases; it also offers a worldwide listing of research and treatment centers.

For a listing of links to Behçet's organizations, specialists and treatment centers around the world, see the file **Docs&Gp** on the CD.

ON THE CD

We've seen in Question 3 that rheumatologists are often the first point of contact for Behçet's patients. The American College of Rheumatology (ACR) has a Geographic Membership Directory, filtered by state or country. It lets you search for a rheumatologist in your area who treats either children or adults. While there's no guarantee this person will be a Behçet's expert, a phone call or email to the specialist's office may get you a referral to a different doctor with more Behçet's experience.

For Behçet's patients worried about their vision, the Ocular Immunology and Uveitis Foundation offers listings of uveitis specialists in the United States and other countries.

You may not have a lot of treatment options if you live in a rural location and/or if you don't have the money to travel for care. If that's the case, ask people in your area to suggest a good primary care doctor who's kind and willing to work together *with* you. It may take a while to find this person (and some people may feel it's impossible), but the rewards can be great if you're able to connect and work well together. How much this doctor knows about Behçet's isn't as important as his or her willingness to learn along with you and to make your health and well-being a priority. Table 1.1 shows what to look for in a good physician or healthcare provider.

"Angel flight" volunteer pilots offer free air transportation for patients who don't have the funds to travel for medical care. You can find local, non-profit angel-flight groups by typing the term "angel flight" into your computer browser's search box.

NOTE

Table 1.1 The traits of a good doctor or other healthcare provider

A good communicator	A good communicator *listens* as well as talks, and pays attention when you speak. He hears your worries and explains medical problems and treatments in plain language so you're able to understand them.

Empathic	He's able to understand your feelings and what you're going through. He can "walk in your shoes."
Professional	He shows respect for your situation and point of view, and he makes it clear your health is his top concern. He's willing to answer questions and talk about any medical information you bring to the appointment. He stays calm even if you don't agree.
Honest	He'll tell you if/when he doesn't know the answer to your question(s). If he's not able to help, he'll find someone else who can.
Attention to detail	He makes sure you get all test results as needed or promised and doesn't make you wait longer for answers than you should.

References

REFERENCES

CHAPTER 1

1. Yazici, H. & Yazici, Y. (Eds.). (2010). *Behçet's Syndrome.* New York, NY: Springer.

2. Kural-Seyahi, E., Fresko, I., Seyahi, N., Ozyazgan, Y., Mat, C., Hamuryudan, V., Yurdakul, S., & Yazici, H. (2003). The long-term mortality and morbidity of Behçet syndrome: a 2-decade outcome survey of 387 patients followed at a dedicated center. *Medicine, 82(1),* 60–76.

3. Hedayatfar, A. (2013). Behçet's Disease: Autoimmune or Autoinflammatory? *Journal of ophthalmic & vision research, 8(3),* 291–293. Available online at http://www.ncbi.nlm.nih.gov/pmc/articles/PMC3853784/pdf/JOVR-08-291.pdf

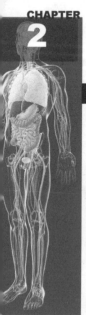

Behçet's disease around the world

5. Where is Behçet's disease most common?

Behçet's disease is linked with the old "Silk Road" trade routes in the Far East, Middle East and Mediterranean (see Figure 2.1). It appears most often between latitudes 30° and 45°N.[3]

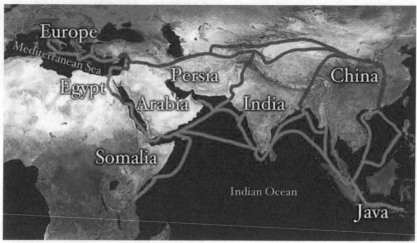

▲ **Figure 2.1**
Land (red) and sea (blue) routes of the Silk Road
Source: http://upload.wikimedia.org/wikipedia/commons/7/74/Silk_route.jpg

Prevalence answers the question "How many people have this disease right now?" The result is usually shown as the number of cases out of every 100,000 people in a country or region. **Incidence** answers the question "How many **new** people develop this disease every year?"

Turkey has the highest prevalence of Behçet's disease in the world: up to 420 people out of every 100,000 people in Turkey have Behçet's. Table 2.1 shows the top ten prevalence rates of Behçet's in countries around the world, from highest rates to lowest. Table 2.2 translates these rates into estimated numbers of Behçet's patients in each country where prevalence rates are available. Table 2.3 shows countries with the highest estimated numbers of Behçet's patients (where Behçet's prevalence rates are available).

Table 2.1 Top ten prevalence rates of Behçet's around the world, from highest to lowest.[4]

Ranking	Country/Region	Prevalence Rate per 100,000 People
1	Turkey	From 80 to 420 cases out of 100,000 people
2	Israel (Druze population)	146
3	Northern China (Ningxiahei)	120
4	Iran	80
5	Germany (Turkish population)	77
6	France (North African population)	35
7	Germany (non-German population)	27
8	Israel (Arab population)	26
9	Saudi Arabia	20
10	Iraq	17

Table 2.2 Estimated numbers of Behçet's patients in countries/regions where prevalence figures are available: Alphabetical by country (from reference [4] unless otherwise specified).

Country/Region	Est. # Behçet's Patients (2014)	Prevalence/100,000 people	Population
Egypt	6,540	7.6	86,048,500
France	4,675	7.1	65,844,000
Germany[12]	580	0.72	80,585,700
Hong Kong	187	2.6	7,184,000
Iran	61,803	80.0	77,254,000
Iraq	5,786	17.0	34,035,000
Israel	1,236	15.2	8,134,000
Italy	2,278	3.8	59,943,933
Japan	17,169	13.5	127,180,000
Kuwait	64	2.1	3,065,850

Country/ Region	Est. # Behçet's Patients (2014)	Prevalence/ 100,000 people	Population
Morocco[11]	4,978	>15	33,188,600
Northern China (Ningxiahei)[10]	7,561	120.0	6,301,350
Portugal	157	1.5	10,487,289
Saudi Arabia	5,999	20.0	29,994,272
Scotland	16	0.3	5,295,000
Spain	2,610 to 3,495	5.6 to 7.5	46,609,700
Sweden	338	3.5	9,644,864
Taiwan	234	1.0	23,377,515
Turkey	61,334 to 322,005	80 to 420	76,667,864
United Kingdom	408[a]	0.64	63,705,000
United States	16,517	5.2	317,635,762

[a] The Behçet's Syndrome Society estimates 1,000 patients in the United Kingdom instead (2013)

Table 2.3 Top ten Behçet's populations in countries/regions where prevalence figures are available.

Ranking	Country/Region	Estimated # Behçet's patients (2014)
1	Turkey	61,334 to 322,005
2	Iran	61,803
3	Japan	17,169
4	United States	16,517
5	Northern China (Ningxiahei)	7,561
6	Egypt	6,540
7	Saudi Arabia	5,999
8	Iraq	5,786
9	Morocco	4,978
10	France	4,675

See a map of the worldwide prevalence of Behçet's disease in file **BDmap** on the CD.

Other countries that have published Behçet's studies or recognized individual or new cases (without giving a prevalence rate) as of 2014 include: Argentina, Australia, Brazil, Canada [author's personal contacts], Chile, Colombia, Cuba, Denmark, Democratic Republic of Congo, French West Indies (Guadeloupe), Greece, Greenland, India, Ireland, Korea, Lebanon, Mexico, Mongolia, Nepal, New Zealand, Norway, Pakistan, Papua New Guinea [author's personal contacts], Poland, Russia, Scotland, South Africa, Taiwan, Thailand, and Venezuela.

6. What about people who move from places where Behçet's is common to places where it isn't?

Research from the Behçet's Syndrome Center in New York City suggests patients in the United States with Silk Road backgrounds might have more severe symptoms than patients who have a Northern European background. Some studies in other countries[4] agree with this view. For example, in Paris, Behçet's is more common in North Africans and Asians living there than in residents who are European natives. In Berlin (a German city with a large, multi-ethnic population), Behçet's appears more often in people with Turkish, Lebanese, or Greek backgrounds than it does in native Germans or people of other ethnicities.[12] In Israel, many more people in the Druze ethno-religious community have Behçet's than other ethnic groups in that country. On the other hand, a 1975 survey of physicians in Hawaii found there were *no* reported cases of Behçet's in the state, even though more than 200,000 Japanese were living there at the time. The prevalence of Behçet's in Japan is 22 cases out of every 100,000 people.

7. Which Behçet's symptoms are most common?

That depends on where you live, because the frequency of some symptoms may vary by country or region. Table 2.4 shows results from research studies done in 26 countries:[1,5]

Table 2.4 Occurrence of Behçet's disease clinical symptoms, from research studies in 26 countries.[a]

Clinical Symptom	% Overall	Country With Highest %	US[5,6]	UK[1]
Oral ulcers	92–100% of BD cases	100% in 12 countries [b]	90–100%	100%
Genital ulcers	62–100% of BD cases	Iraq (100%)	62–73%	89%
Skin lesions	39–90% of BD cases	Jordan (90%)	67–85%	86%
Eye involvement	29–92% of BD cases	Italy (92%)	27–70%	68%
Joint involvement	16–94% of BD cases	France (94%)	46–51%	93%
CNS involvement	2–44% of BD cases	Saudi Arabia (44%)	16–23%	31%
GI involvement	3–37% of BD cases	Russia (37%)	34%	7%
Phlebitis	5–37% of BD cases	Russia (37%)	4%	22%
Epididymitis	1–28% of BD cases	Jordan (28%)	1%	--

[a] Iran, Japan, China, Korea, Germany, Turkey, Morocco, Tunisia, United Kingdom, India, Saudi Arabia, Iraq, Jordan, Lebanon, Israel, Egypt, Algeria, Tadjikistan, Russia, Greece, Italy, Portugal, France, United States, Brazil, Spain
[b] Turkey, Morocco, Tunisia, United Kingdom, Saudi Arabia, Iraq, Jordan, Tadjikistan, Russia, Greece, Brazil, Spain

Some Behçet's patients have **symptom clusters.** For example, acne (in patients not on corticosteroids), arthritis and enthesopathy (abnormalities in places where tendons, ligaments and/or muscles join to the bone) often occur at the same time. Another symptom cluster is deep vein thrombosis (DVT), superficial venous thrombosis (SVT) and dural sinus thrombosis. Eighty percent of patients with pulmonary artery aneurysms (PAA) also have peripheral DVT.[7]

NOTE

8. How is Behçet's in the United States and Western/ Northern Europe different from Behçet's in Silk Road countries?

Historically, more men than women have Behçet's in parts of the world where the disease is common. More women than men have had Behçet's, though, in Northern Europe and the United States.[1] However, these trends seem to be changing: there are now almost equal numbers of men and women with Behçet's in the United Kingdom, which is the same as results coming in from other European and Turkish studies.[2] Recent published work from Hatemi and the Yazicis (2013)[7] agrees.

Table 2.5 shows some other differences between Behçet's patients in the United States and Northern and Western Europe, and those along the Silk Road.

Table 2.5 Differences between Behçet's patients in the US/Northern and Western Europe, and along the Silk Road.[4,5,6]

US / Northern and Western Europe	Silk Road
Traditionally more women than men	Traditionally more men than women
Positive pathergy results in ~20% of patients	Positive pathergy results in ~50% of patients
~15% of patients are HLA-B51 positive; 49% of US BD patients with Northern European descent positive for HLA-DRB1*04 in 1998 O'Duffy study[9]	50–80% of patients are HLA-B51 positive
Often milder disease course, with more females, skin and mucous membrane symptoms	More severe disease in young, male, Middle/Far Eastern patients

References

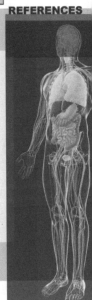

CHAPTER 2

1. Davatchi, F., Shahram, F., Chams-Davatchi, C., Shams, H., Nadji, A., Akhlaghi, M.,...Sadeghi Abdollahi, B. (2010). Behcet's disease: from East to West. *Clinical rheumatology, 29(8),* 823–833. Available online at http://www.ncbi.nlm.nih.gov/pubmed/20354748

2. Russell, A. I., Lawson, W. A., & Haskard, D. O. (2001). Potential new therapeutic options in Behcet's syndrome. *BioDrugs: clinical immunotherapeutics, biopharmaceuticals and gene therapy, 15(1),* 25–35.

3. Cho, S. B., Cho, S., & Bang, D. (2012). New insights in the clinical understanding of Behçet's disease. *Yonsei medical journal, 53(1)*, 35–42. Available online at http://dx.doi.org/10.3349/ymj.2012.53.1.35

4. Yurdakul, S. & Yazici, Y. (2010). Epidemiology of Behçet's syndrome and regional differences in disease expression. In Yazici, H. & Yazici, Y. (Eds.), *Behçet's Syndrome*. (pp. 35-52). New York, NY: Springer.

5. Kobayashi, T., Kishimoto, M., Swearingen, C. J., Filopoulos, M. T., Ohara, Y., Tokuda, Y.... Yazici, Y. (2013). Differences in clinical manifestations, treatment, and concordance rates with two major sets of criteria for Behçet's syndrome for patients in the US and Japan: data from a large, three-center cohort study. *Modern rheumatology / the Japan Rheumatism Association, 23(3)*, 547–553.

6. Calamia, K. T., Wilson, F. C., Icen, M., Crowson, C. S., Gabriel, S. E., & Kremers, H. M. (2009). Epidemiology and clinical characteristics of Behçet's disease in the US: a population-based study. *Arthritis and rheumatism, 61(5)*, 600–604. Available online at http://www.ncbi.nlm.nih.gov/pmc/articles/PMC3024036/pdf/nihms258832.pdf

7. Hatemi, G., Yazici, Y., & Yazici, H. (2013). Behçet's syndrome. *Rheumatic disease clinics of North America, 39(2)*, 245–261.

8. Calamia, K. T. (June 2002). Behcet's disease: the USA scene. International Society for Behçet's Disease. *BD News, 3*(1), 1-3. Article available online at http://behcet.ws/behcetwsData/Document/1662014135413-v3.pdf

9. O'Duffy, J. D., Tirzaman, O., Weyand, C. M., & Goronzy, J. J. (1998, October). HLA-DRB1 alleles in Behçet's disease (Abstract P17). *Proceedings of the Eighth International Congress on Behçet's disease*, Reggio-Emilia, Italy, p.113.

10. Kaneko, F., Nakamura, K., Sato, M., Tojo, M., Zheng, X., & Zhang, J. Z. (2003). Epidemiology of Behçet's disease in Asian countries and Japan. *Advances in experimental medicine and biology, 528*, 25–29.

11. Verity, D. H., Marr, J. E., Ohno, S., Wallace, G. R., & Stanford, M. R. (1999). Behçet's disease, the Silk Road and HLA-B51: historical and geographical perspectives. *Tissue antigens, 54(3)*, 213–220.

12. Papoutsis, N. G., Abdel-Naser, M. B., Altenburg, A., Orawa, H., Kötter, I., Krause, L.,... Zouboulis, C. C. (2006). Prevalence of Adamantiades-Behçet's disease in Germany and the municipality of Berlin: results of a nationwide survey. *Clinical and experimental rheumatology, 24(5 Suppl 42)*, S125. Available online at http://www.clinexprheumatol.org/pubmed/find-pii.asp?pii=17067445

Diagnosis of Behçet's disease

9. Is there any test that will definitely prove you have Behçet's disease?

No, there is no diagnostic test for Behçet's. A Behçet's diagnosis is based on a patient's signs, symptoms and prognosis (how a disease will probably act over time), and it's given after all other diagnostic options have been ruled out. Conditions that have some symptoms similar to Behçet's include celiac disease, erythema multiforme, hand-foot-mouth disease, hematological diseases (such as cyclic neutropenia and lymphoma), herpes simplex, Hughes–Stovin syndrome, inflammatory bowel disease (such as Crohn's and ulcerative colitis), lupus, Lyme disease, MAGIC syndrome, mixed connective tissue diseases, multiple sclerosis, mucous membrane pemphigus, nutritional deficiencies (iron, B12, folic acid), psoriatic arthritis, recurrent aphthous stomatitis, Reiter's syndrome, sarcoidosis, Stevens-Johnson syndrome and Sweet's syndrome. It's also possible for Behçet's to overlap, or happen at the same time, as any of these illnesses. As a result, it's not surprising that it can take months or years for some patients to be diagnosed.

What's the difference between a symptom and a sign?
According to CommunicateHealth.com, a *symptom* is something only you know is there. A *sign* is something other people (like your doctor) can notice.

10. What types of test results are common (but not required) when trying to diagnose Behçet's?

Some abnormal test results may show up more often in Behçet's patients than in healthy people, but these results can show up in people with other illnesses, too—not just Behçet's. It's also possible to get a Behçet's diagnosis without having *any* abnormal lab or blood test results: that's why lab and blood tests aren't foolproof ways to diagnose BD. If results are abnormal, though, they may help some

Read an article that gives in-depth information on illnesses with Behçet's-like symptoms: *Clinical and pathological manifestations with differential diagnosis in Behçet's disease* (2012) at http://downloads.hindawi.com/journals/pri/2012/690390.pdf

patients show their doctors that they have a good reason for feeling poorly.

Here is a summary of some abnormal lab and blood test results in Behçet's patients:[1]

- CRP and ESR levels (measures of inflammation in the body) are sometimes—*but not always*—significantly higher in patients with active Behçet's than they are in healthy people, or in BD patients with no symptoms. People with normal CRP and ESR levels can still receive a BD diagnosis, though, based on other relevant signs and symptoms.
- IL-6, IL-8, TNF, serum beta 2-microglobulin, serum amyloid A protein, and/or mean C_3 and C_4 levels *may* be higher in patients with active Behçet's than in healthy people.

11. What is a pathergy test and is it necessary for diagnosis?

A positive pathergy test result can often *help* diagnose a case of Behçet's, but a positive result isn't *required* for diagnosis. (See Question 15 on Classification Criteria for Behçet's.)

Many Behçet's patients have an over-the-top, hyper-reactive skin response to scratches or other injuries. This response is called *pathergy*. A pathergy test is when a doctor pricks a patient's forearm in three places with a sterile needle to see if a pustule (a small, raised, inflamed area of skin filled with lymph fluid or pus) forms at the site within 24–48 hours. Requirements for the pathergy test appear in Question 15. Only one of the three skin pricks needs to show a reaction in order to say the test result is positive. A 2002 study found significant results by pricking the inside of the patient's lower lip instead. This technique is not as sensitive as the forearm test, but the results are easier to read because they look like regular BD oral lesions.[13] In 2011, researchers found that pricking a BD patient's forearm with the patient's own saliva also created a positive reaction (a red area bigger than 10mm, or pustules bigger than 2mm after 24 hours) in 9 out of 10 participants.[14]

Behçet's patients in the United States and Northern/Western Europe hardly ever have positive pathergy test results, even if they have active symptoms and a firm Behçet's diagnosis. Even in Middle Eastern and Far Eastern countries, the frequency of positive results has been dropping. For example, positive pathergy results in Iranian Behçet's patients have dropped from 61% of BD patients before

1977 to 41% as of 2007. Why the change? It may be due to doctors switching to thin, disposable sterile needles for the test, and steering away from older blunt needles that may have caused more skin trauma and inflammation (and positive results). Doing a thorough skin cleansing before the test, or using antibiotic cream afterwards on the test sites, can also lower the number of positive results.[4] Taking corticosteroids like prednisone at the time of the test can have the same effect.[3]

Instead of using a pathergy test to help with diagnosis, some physicians look for pathergy "equivalents" in their patients: skin bumps or lumps where needles were inserted for acupuncture or an EMG test; eye inflammation/uveitis after a cataract has been removed, or after injections of corticosteroids into the eye; a blood clot, superficial thrombophlebitis, or pustule at the site of an IV insertion, blood draw or skin trauma; or new intestinal ulcers that appear at the surgical treatment site of intestinal ulceration(s).[4,6]

12. What is an HLA test?

HLA stands for *human leukocyte antigen*. HLA blood tests are often used for genetic counseling and to check if an organ donor matches an organ recipient. Your HLA types are inherited from both sides of your family, and they don't change, just like your blood type doesn't change. A sample of your blood is all that's needed to get your HLA types. Your doctor will send your blood to the lab and ask for a list of all HLA-A, -B, -C, or -D types that show up in your blood. Getting these results can be expensive, though, and if you live in the United States, testing may not be covered by your health insurance. It may also take weeks for your results to arrive.

Researchers have linked the following HLA types with Behçet's disease: HLA-B5, HLA-B51, HLA-DRB1, and HLA-A26.[4,6] Even if you have one of these HLA types, though, it doesn't mean you definitely have Behçet's: 10–20% of healthy people are positive for HLA-B5 too, but they never develop BD.[15] More information can be found at Question 15.

13. Do you need a positive HLA-B5 or HLA-B51 test result to get a Behçet's diagnosis?

No. Diagnosis comes when a doctor who's very familiar with Behçet's goes over your medical history, looks at your signs and hears about your symptoms, does tests to rule out other illnesses, and uses his/her knowledge of BD patients and Behçet's criteria to make an informed decision (see Question 15). While many Behçet's patients—especially in the Silk Road countries—may have positive HLA-B5 or HLA-B51 results, many other formally diagnosed BD patients **don't** have those results.

14. Does a positive HLA-B5 or HLA-B51 result mean you'll have a worse case of Behçet's?

Not necessarily. A 2012 review of 74 research studies from 24 countries[7] found that a positive HLA-B51 or HLA-B5 result appears slightly more often in male Behçet's patients and is linked to a higher risk of genital ulcers, skin lesions, and eye involvement. It's also linked to a *lower* risk of gastrointestinal involvement. People with positive HLA-B51 or -B5 results don't seem to have a higher risk of major blood vessel involvement or central nervous system disease, which are two of the most serious Behçet's complications. Some other research results don't agree with these findings, though: they suggest that HLA-B51 *is* a marker of a worse case of Behçet's.[8,9] All of these results are just an overview of the topic, since most of the studies have taken place in Silk Road countries. Your own situation (and location) may be different.

15. What are "Classification Criteria for Behçet's"?

Classification Criteria for Behçet's were originally set up to help researchers choose BD patients who were similar to each other for research studies. There have been at least 15 different sets of Behçet's criteria, dating back to 1946. The 1990 International Study Group (ISG) criteria are the most familiar to researchers and rheumatologists; they're also the most widely used (see Table 3.1).

Table 3.1 International Study Group (ISG) Classification Criteria for Behçet's Disease

Recurrent oral ulcerations (required)	a. Minor aphthous ulceration b. Major aphthous or herpetiform ulceration observed by a physician or reported reliably by patient c. Recurrent at least 3x in a 12-month period

Plus TWO of the following:	
Recurrent genital ulcerations	Recurrent genital aphthous ulceration or scarring, especially males, observed by physician or reliably reported by patient
Eye lesions	a. Anterior uveitis b. Posterior uveitis c. Cells in vitreous on slit lamp examination **or** d. Retinal vasculitis observed by ophthalmologist
Skin lesions	a. Erythema-nodosum-like lesions observed by physician or reliably reported by patient b. Pseudofolliculitis c. Papulopustular lesions **or** d. Acneiform nodules consistent with Behçet's disease, observed by a physician, and in post-adolescent patients not receiving corticosteroids
Positive pathergy test	An erythematous papule, >2mm, at the prick site 48 hours after the application of a sterile needle, 20–22 gauge, which obliquely penetrates avascular skin to a depth of 5mm: read by physician at 48 hours.

International Criteria for Behçet's Disease (ICBD)

The older ISG criteria have some shortcomings. For example, according to the ISG, all Behçet's patients must have oral ulcers to get a diagnosis, even though a small number of properly diagnosed patients may never have them. As a result, new criteria have been proposed and are still being tested under the name "International Criteria for Behçet's Disease" (ICBD). Twenty-seven countries provided patient data to create the ICBD. There's no time estimate when—or if—these newer criteria will be officially adopted.

Under the scoring system for the ICBD, a Behçet's diagnosis is a total score that's greater than or equal to 4 (see Table 3.2). A 2013 article about the ICBD[11] gives a little more detail about the diagnosis if a patient's total is 4 or greater (not including pathergy results): a total of 4 is "probably BD," a 5 is "highly likely BD," and a 6 or higher is "almost certainly BD." Any point total less than 4 is not considered to be Behçet's. In countries where Behçet's is rare, it's important for a Behçet's-experienced doctor to look at a patient's full signs, symptoms, medical history and test results to decide on a diagnosis, and not rely on any particular set of criteria.

Table 3.2 Scoring system for International Criteria for Behçet's Disease (ICBD). A total score of 4 or higher provides a Behçet's diagnosis.

Point value	Sign/symptom	Description
2 points	Ocular lesions Genital aphthous ulcers Oral aphthous ulcers	**Anterior uveitis, posterior uveitis** or **retinal vasculitis**
1 point	Skin lesions	Pseudofolliculitis, aphthous skin ulcers or erythema nodosum
	Neurological issues	Does **not** include headaches unless they're due to other serious neurological problems (for example, aseptic meningitis or intracranial hypertension)
	Vascular issues	Arterial thrombosis, large vein thrombosis, phlebitis or superficial phlebitis
	Positive pathergy test result – OPTIONAL, but worth 1 point if present when tested	

Here's a scoring example: A patient has 10 oral aphthous ulcers (2 points), had erythema nodosum two months ago (1 point) and has ongoing retinal vasculitis (2 points). This patient has a total of 5 points, which not only means a Behçet's diagnosis, but one that's "highly likely." However, some experts feel a total score and diagnosis should also be tied to a patient's ethnic background or where he lives. In other words, a patient who lives in a Silk Road country may be considered "highly likely" or "almost certainly" to have a BD diagnosis with a point total of only 4. A Northern/Western European native, though, may need to reach a total of 5 or 6 before getting a definite BD diagnosis from some doctors.

16. Should doctors use Classification Criteria to diagnose Behçet's patients?

There's a split between Behçet's experts on whether *any* Behçet's Classification Criteria should be used to diagnose individual patients. Some experts feel criteria should only exist to put patients in groups for research studies; diagnosis is best left to Behçet's specialists who understand the disease and its effects on all body systems. Other experts, like the Yazici father–son team, say "Diagnosis is nothing more or less than a classification for the individual patient."[10] According to Kenneth Calamia, MD (personal communication): "The diagnosis in any individual is based on knowledgeable clinical judgment, taking into consideration multiple things not included in criteria, such as age, gender, [specific] vascular, neurologic, and GI manifestations, the presence of manifestations that should not be part of the disease, and the presence of other diseases which could cause similar symptoms or findings."

Since experienced Behçet's specialists aren't always available for diagnosis, though, physicians should be able to use Behçet's Classification Criteria as a strong diagnostic aid. It could help many patients begin treatment sooner and possibly avoid some of the more severe complications of untreated Behçet's.

17. Do you need to show all of the standard Behçet's symptoms *at the same time* to get a Behçet's diagnosis?

No. As long as Behçet's signs/symptoms are documented over time through pictures, test results and/or notes in the patient's medical record, it's not necessary for a doctor to see all of the important symptoms during a single scheduled appointment.

18. Can you get a Behçet's diagnosis even if you live in countries where it isn't common, like the United States or the United Kingdom?

Yes, but it may not be easy. Some North American and Western European physicians still believe that only people from the Middle East should get a Behçet's diagnosis. However, Behçet's experts know the disease is found worldwide, regardless of a person's known ethnic background or birthplace. Once other possible causes for BD-type symptoms have been ruled out, Behçet's becomes the best diagnosis.

REFERENCES

References

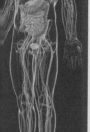

CHAPTER 3

1. Melikoglu, M., & Topkarci, Z. (2014). Is there a relation between clinical disease activity and acute phase response in Behcet's disease? *International journal of dermatology,53(2)*, 250–254.

2. Yazici, Y., Erkan, D., Ince, A., Nesher, G., Kural, E., Seyahi, N., & Moore, T. L. (2004). Behçet's disease: does lack of knowledge result in under-diagnosis? *Clinical and experimental rheumatology, 22(4 Suppl 34)*, 81–82.

3. Davatchi, F., Chams-Davatchi, C., Ghodsi, Z., Shahram, F., Nadji, A., Shams, H...& Sadeghi-Abdolahi, B. (2011). Diagnostic value of pathergy test in Behcet's disease according to the change of incidence over the time. *Clinical rheumatology, 30(9)*, 1151–1155.

4. Barnes, C. (2010) History and Diagnosis. In Yazici, H. & Yazici, Y. (Eds.), *Behçet's Syndrome* (pp. 7-34). New York, NY: Springer.

5. Davatchi, F., Chams-Davatchi, C., Ghodsi, Z., Shahram, F., Nadji, A., Shams, H., Akhlaghi, M., Larimi, R., & Sadeghi-Abdolahi, B. (2011). Diagnostic value of pathergy test in Behcet's disease according to the change of incidence over the time. *Clinical rheumatology, 30(9)*, 1151–1155.

6. Calamia, K. (May 12–15, 2011). Congress of Clinical Rheumatology: Update on Behcet's Disease in the USA.

7. Maldini, C., Lavalley, M. P., Cheminant, M., de Menthon, M., & Mahr, A. (2012). Relationships of HLA-B51 or B5 genotype with Behcet's disease clinical characteristics: systematic review and meta-analyses of observational studies. *Rheumatology (Oxford, England), 51(5)*, 887–900.

8. Zouboulis, C.C. (1999). Epidemiology of Adamantiades- Behcet's disease. *Annales de médecine interne, 150*(6), 488-498.

9. Chang, H. K., Kim, J. U., Cheon, K. S., Chung, H. R., Lee, K. W., & Lee, I. H. (2001). HLA-B51 and its allelic types in association with Behçet's disease and recurrent aphthous stomatitis in Korea. *Clinical and experimental rheumatology, 19(5 Suppl 24)*, S31-5.

10. Hatemi, G., Yazici, Y., & Yazici, H. (2013). Behçet's syndrome. *Rheumatic disease clinics of North America, 39(2)*, 245–261.

11. International Team for the Revision of the International Criteria for Behçet's Disease (64 members). (2014). The International Criteria for Behçet's Disease (ICBD): a collaborative study of 27 countries on the sensitivity and specificity of the new criteria. *Journal of the European Academy of Dermatology and Venereology: JEADV, 28(3)*, 338–347.

12. E. A. Graykowski, M. F. Barile, W. B. Lee, & H. R. Stanley Jr. (1966). Recurrent aphthous stomatitis. Clinical, therapeutic, histopathologic, and hypersensitivity aspects. *The Journal of the American Medical Association, 196*(7), 637–644.

13. Sharquie, K. E., Al-Araji, A., & Hatem, A. (2002). Oral pathergy test in Behçet's disease. *The British journal of dermatology, 146(1)*, 168–169.

14. Togashi, A., Saito, S., Kaneko, F., Nakamura, K., & Oyama, N. (2011). Skin prick test with self-saliva in patients with oral aphthoses: a diagnostic pathergy for Behcet's disease and recurrent aphthosis. *Inflammation & Allergy Drug Targets, 10(3)*, 164–170. Available online at http://www.ncbi.nlm.nih.gov/pmc/articles/PMC3228232/pdf/IADT-10-164.pdf

15. Kalra, S., Silman, A., Akman-Demir, G., Bohlega, S., Borhani-Haghighi, A., Constantinescu...Siva, A., & Al-Araji, A. (2013). Diagnosis and management of neuro-Behçet's disease: international consensus recommendations. *Journal of neurology, Published online 24 December 2013*. Available at http://link.springer.com/article/10.1007%2Fs00415-013-7209-3

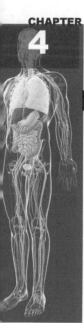

Oral and genital sores and other skin lesions

19. Does everyone with Behçet's get mouth ulcers?

No. As many as three out of every 100 properly-diagnosed Behçet's patients have never had mouth sores (oral aphthous ulcers). Doctors who understand how Behçet's affects the different systems of the body can often recognize BD patients even if they never have oral ulcers. Healthcare providers who don't have much experience with Behçet's, though, may have a problem diagnosing a patient who doesn't have mouth sores: that's because the International Study Group (ISG) Classification Criteria for Behçet's—which many doctors use to help diagnose a case of BD—say that oral lesions have to show up at least three times in 12 months. The newer International Criteria for Behçet's Disease (ICBD), still being tested, looks at oral ulcers differently by saying they're no longer required for diagnosis. This approach allows for an earlier diagnosis and treatment for people who may not receive it otherwise—especially since it may take months or years for all "required" ISG BD symptoms to show up for a firm diagnosis. See Question 15 for more information on the ICBD and other Behçet's criteria.

20. What types of skin lesions can be caused by Behçet's, and what do they look like?

Many different types of skin lesions are listed in the ISG Classification Criteria for Behçet's: oral aphthous ulcers, genital aphthous ulcers, erythema nodosum, pseudofolliculitis, papulopustular lesions, and acneiform nodules in adult patients who aren't taking prednisone or other corticosteroids. Here is more information on each one:

- **Oral aphthous** (app-thus) **ulcers** look like regular canker sores that ulcerate (see Figure 4.1). They often appear years before any other Behçet's symptoms, but recurrent canker sores can also show up in 20% of people who *never* develop BD. These oral ulcers may be so painful that patients have trouble eating and speaking, especially if several ulcers appear in the mouth at once. Typical ulcer locations include the inside lining of the cheeks, the inside of the lips where they touch the teeth, the tongue, gums, and the back of the roof of the mouth. An ulcer may start after this mucosal skin inside the mouth has been injured or scratched, although some BD-related oral ulcers can also appear on their own with no advance injuries. These ulcers aren't contagious and come in three types: *minor*, which are the most common (<10 mm in diameter; < 3/8") and often heal in 7–10 days without scarring; *major* (>10 mm in diameter), which may take two to four weeks or more to heal and may leave scars; and *herpetiform*—large crops of very small ulcers that appear in one part of the mouth; they sometimes join together into a big ulcerated area that may leave a scar and takes weeks to heal. In spite of the name, herpetiform ulcers are not caused by the herpes virus.

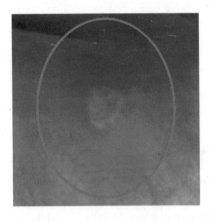

◄ **Figure 4.1**
An oral aphthous ulcer
Source: http://commons.wikimedia.org/wiki/
File:Aphthe_Unterlippe.jpg

- **Genital aphthous ulcers** are usually painful and look like oral aphthous ulcers, with their typical punched-out appearance. They start as tender red lumps or pustules, like a whitehead, that eventually ulcerate. They usually heal in two to four weeks, but it may take longer if several ulcers have fused together into a large ulcerated area. Healing time will also be extended if the ulcers become infected. Not every Behçet's patient gets genital ulcers, and they're not required for diagnosis if the patient has other relevant symptoms listed in the ISG Classification Criteria. In males, these ulcers appear most often on the scrotum, but they can also show up on the tip of the penis and the shaft. In females, lesions can be on the labia, in the vagina—where they may cause a discharge—and/or on the cervix. Some of the author's personal Behçet's contacts (women) have reported getting tender, red genital lumps that don't always ulcerate.

In both sexes, genital ulcers can show up in the groin, around the anus (perianal region) or between the vagina and anus or the scrotum and anus (the perineal region). Genital ulcers may leave scars.

- **Erythema nodosum-like lesions** are tender, raised red nodules (solid lumps in or under the skin) that usually appear on the lower legs or shins, but they can also be on the neck, face, forearms, thighs, ankles and buttocks (see Image 4.2). They are often 1–3 cm (3/8"-1 ¼") in size, and they don't usually ulcerate. They typically last from one to six weeks and may sometimes leave behind areas that look like bruises.

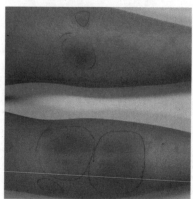

◀ **Figure 4.2**
Erythema nodosum
Source: http://commons.wikimedia.org/wiki/File:ENlegs.JPG

- **Pseudofolliculitis, papulopustular lesions, and acneiform nodules** are all listed together as one symptom category in the ISG Criteria for Behçet's (see Question 15) to help with diagnosis. In a 1997 article, Lee, Bank & Lee admit that "The terms are very confusing"[1] because—in many ways—these lesions look similar to each other. In fact, it may be hard for even skilled clinicians to tell them apart. In general, though, *pseudofolliculitis* (see Figure 4.3) is an inflammation of hair follicles, sometimes looking like a rash of whiteheads on the back, shoulders or other areas. *Papulopustular lesions* are solid, red, raised areas on the skin that may be filled with pus or clear lymph fluid, although this fluid may or may not be visible from the outside. A 2012 article[2] found that people with BD who get papulopustular lesions also tend to have arthritis and joint involvement. *Acneiform nodules* may look like ordinary acne, with inflamed papules, pustules or nodules. Experts feel that young adults and people taking corticosteroids may have age- and/or medication-related acne instead of Behçet's acneiform nodules. People with Behçet's-related nodules get them more often on their body, including their arms and legs, than on their face and neck.

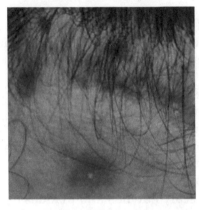

◀ **Figure 4.3**
Pseudofolliculitis
Source: http://commons.wikimedia.
org/wiki/File:Folliculitis_at_the_
back_of_hair_scalp_which_also_
spread_to_upper_part_of_the_
back_body.jpeg

- **Superficial thrombophlebitis** is the hard, painful inflammation of a vein just under the skin's surface, in places where the vein has been injured or where an IV line has been inserted.
- **Extragenital ulcerations** look like typical Behçet's oral/genital ulcers, but they show up in other places. Researchers have seen these lesions on the breasts, legs, feet, groin area, armpits and necks of Behçet's patients.[4] Extragenital ulcers often leave scars.

Other types of skin lesions reported in BD patients[3] can help with diagnosis, but only when doctors who have experience with Behçet's add them to a patient's overall signs/symptoms, full medical history and test results. These other lesions include:

ON THE WEB See more pictures of different types of Behçet's skin lesions in these two articles: *Dermatologic Manifestation of Behçet's Disease* at http://www.eymj.org/Synapse/Data/PDFData/0069YMJ/ymj-38-380.pdf and *Mucocutaneous Lesions of Behçet's Disease* at http://www.ncbi.nlm.nih.gov/pmc/articles/PMC2628050/

- *Leg ulcers*: lesions on the leg that may resist treatment and are often caused by vasculitis or deep vein thrombosis
- *Cellulitis*: an infection that spreads to deeper tissues, often on the legs, arms, or face. The area looks warm,

red, swollen, and tender. See your doctor right away if this area grows or extends red streaks

- *Erythema multiforme-like lesion*: a dark red elevated area on the skin, sometimes having a ringed "target" appearance
- *Nodule*: a usually painless, solid and raised area in or under the skin
- *Vesicle or bulla*: a clear fluid-filled blister on the skin. A vesicle can be up to about 1cm in size (a little more than 3/8") and a bulla is larger than 1cm. *Bullae* is the plural of bulla
- *Pyoderma*: a bacterial skin inflammation that comes on suddenly and is filled with pus
- *Abscess*: a collection of pus inside infected tissue
- *Impetigo*: an inflammatory skin disease with pustules that crust over and rupture
- *Furuncle*: a boil or infected hair follicle
- *Psoriasis*: red and white scaly patches and plaques of skin that usually itch
- *Purpura*: hemorrhaged areas under the skin that may look red at first, darkening into purple; they don't turn white when pressed
- *Urticaria*: hives
- *Eczema*: patches of red to brownish-gray skin that itch. Skin may be thick, scaly, or cracked, with areas of small raised bumps. Scratching the bumps releases fluid that crusts over, and may lead to a skin infection
- *Paronychia*[9]: redness and swelling where the nail and skin meet, along the side or base of a toenail or fingernail (see Figure 4.4)

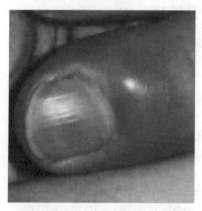

◄ **Figure 4.4**
Paronychia
Source: http://commons.wikimedia.org/wiki/File:Paronychia.jpg

Many personal Behçet's contacts also report small, individual, extremely itchy and painful blisters that are filled with clear fluid. They usually appear on or between the fingers, on the feet/ankles/toes, or as single lesions on other parts of the body. Similar small, painful lesions have also been reported on the scalp.

21. Are there over-the-counter or prescribed medications to help with prevention, pain and/or healing of these ulcers?

Yes, and you should be able to get treatment from your doctor(s) even if you don't have a Behçet's diagnosis. Here are some available options for pain control and/or healing of oral and genital ulcers.[3] **(P = prescription needed in the United States.)** Other treatments are listed in Chapter 13. Some of these treatments may have different names outside the United States.

- **Oral ulcers**

  Local anesthetics to help with pain: Anbesol; Blistex Kanka mouth pain liquid; Canker Cover patches; Iglu mouth ulcer gel; Orabase; Oragel; Topex topical anesthetic gel (benzocaine 20%); Zilactin mouth sore gel; Cetacaine topical metered spray **(P)**; Lidex gel 0.05% (fluocinonide) **(P)**; Lidocaine Viscous 2% **(P)**

  Other treatments: Carmex ointment; Dr. Tichenor's antiseptic mouthwash diluted 3:1; Aphthasol (amlexanox) 5% paste **(P)**; Carafate (sucralfate) Suspension **(P)**; colchicine **(P)**; Dapsone **(P)**; Difflam NSAID mouth rinse (reduces pain and inflammation) **(P)**; Ergamisol (levamisole) **(P)**; Interferon-alpha injections **(P)**; Kenalog in Orabase (triamcinolone) **(P)**; **Magic Mouthwash** or **Bilson's Solution (P)**; penicillin, or penicillin and colchicine **(P)**; Peridex antibacterial mouth rinse (chlorhexidine gluconate 0.12%) **(P)**; prednisone **(P)**; tetracycline dissolved in water as a mouth rinse **(P)**; Trental (pentoxifylline) **(P)**; triamcinolone acetonide injections at the base of ulcers; and Thalomid (thalidomide) **(P)**.

ON THE WEB

For detailed information on dosage amounts for drugs in this section, see the following articles: *Mucocutaneous Lesions of Behçet's Disease* at http://www.ncbi.nlm.nih.gov/pmc/articles/PMC2628050/ (pages 581-2) and *Ulcerative Lesions in Behçet's Disease* at http://www.hindawi.com/journals/ulcers/2012/146797/ (pages 4-7).

- **Genital ulcers**

  Local anesthetics: Vagisil; Baby Orajel with a covering of Vaseline prior to urinating; Liquidcaine; ELA-Max 5 (5% lidocaine) **(P)**; EMLA cream **(P)**; Instillagel (Clinimed) – Canada/UK only **(P)**; Lidex gel (fluocinomide) **(P)**; Sustaine Blue Gel Lidocaine Viscous 2% **(P)**

  Other treatments: Preparation H; urinating while in a shower/bath and spraying the area with a hand-held water spray; Bactroban antibacterial ointment (mupirocin) **(P)**; CellCept (mycophenolate mofetil) **(P)**; colchicine **(P)**; cyclosporine **(P)**; Dapsone **(P)**; Elocon cream/ointment (anti-inflammatory corticosteroid) **(P)**; Enbrel (etanercept) **(P)**; Ergamisol (levamisole) **(P)**; Imuran (azathioprine) **(P)**; interferon alpha-2A **(P)**; Kenacomb cream/ointment (antibacterial/anti-inflammatory) **(P)**; Kenalog in Orabase (triamcinolone) **(P)**; methotrexate **(P)**; Mycolog cream/ointment (antifungal steroidal cream) **(P)**; Peridex antibacterial rinse applied genitally **(P)**; prednisone **(P)**; Remicade (infliximab) **(P)**; Sigmacort (hydrocortisone acetate; topical corticosteroid) **(P)**; sucralfate (topical) **(P)**; Thalomid (thalidomide) **(P)**; Trental (pentoxifylline) **(P)**; triamcinolone injections at the base of stubborn ulcers

Notes about other treatment options

- Genital-area ulcerations may get infected with bacteria. Use antiseptics and antimicrobials on the skin as prescribed by your doctor.
- The drug apremilast (Otezla) may offer safe and effective treatment for Behçet's patients who have oral and genital ulcers. Otezla received FDA approval in early 2014 to treat psoriatic arthritis, but its use in Behçet's patients is still off-label and in clinical trials. This status may change after 2014.
- Some cigarette smokers have developed oral ulcers after they've quit smoking, leading researchers to wonder if nicotine could slow or stop the development of aphthous ulcers. In a very small 2010 study, Behçet's patients who were ex-smokers tried using nicotine patches to get rid of their oral and/or genital lesions.[8] All patches were applied according to nicotine patch instructions, *not* directly on the ulcers themselves. While the patches worked on four out of five patients, lesions returned once their use was stopped.

References

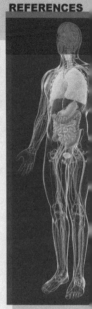

CHAPTER 4

1. Lee, E. S., Bang, D., & Lee, S. (1997). Dermatologic manifestation of Behçet's disease. *Yonsei medical journal, 38(6),* 380–389. Available online at http://www.eymj.org/Synapse/Data/PDFData/0069YMJ/ymj-38-380.pdf

2. Karaca, M., Hatemi, G., Sut, N., & Yazici, H. (2012). The papulopustular lesion/arthritis cluster of Behçet's syndrome also clusters in families. *Rheumatology (Oxford, England), 51(6),* 1053–1060. Available online at http://rheumatology.oxfordjournals.org/content/51/6/1053.full.pdf+html

3. Zeis, J. (2003). *Essential Guide to Behçet's Disease.* Central Vision Press, Uxbridge, MA.

4. Azizlerli, G., Ozarmağan, G., Ovül, C., Sarica, R., & Mustafa, S. O. (1992). A new kind of skin lesion in Behçet's disease: extragenital ulcerations. *Acta dermato-venereologica, 72(4),* 286.

5. Alpsoy, E., Zouboulis, C. C., & Ehrlich, G. E. (2007). Mucocutaneous lesions of Behcet's disease. *Yonsei medical journal, 48(4),* 573–585. Available online at http://www.ncbi.nlm.nih.gov/pmc/articles/PMC2628050

6. Mat, M. C., Bang, D., & Melikoglu, M. (2010). The mucocutaneous manifestations and pathergy reaction in Behçet's Disease. In Yazici, H. & Yazici, Y. (Eds.), *Behçet's Syndrome* (pp. 53–72). New York, NY: Springer.

7. Türsen, U. & Türsen, B. (2012). Ulcerative Lesions in Behcet's Disease. *Ulcers,* vol. 2012, Article ID 146797, 1-9, Accessed at http://www.hindawi.com/journals/ulcers/2012/146797/

8. Ciancio, G., Colina, M., La Corte, R., Lo Monaco, A., De Leonardis, F., Trotta, F., & Govoni, M. (2010). Nicotine-patch therapy on mucocutaneous lesions of Behçet's disease: a case series. *Rheumatology (Oxford, England), 49(3),* 501–504. Available online at http://rheumatology.oxfordjournals.org/content/49/3/501.full.pdf+html

9. Plotkin, G. R., Calabro, J. J., & O'Duffy, J. D. (Eds.) (1998). *Behcet's Disease: A Contemporary Synopsis.* Chapter 12: Miscellaneous Clinical Manifestations. II. Mount Kisco, New York: Futura Publishing Company.

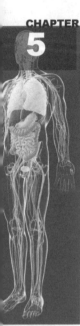

Eye disease in Behçet's

22. What types of eye problems can happen with Behçet's?[1,2,3,4]

In general, three out of every four Behçet's patients eventually develop eye problems. These problems often affect the uveal tract, which is the middle layer of the eye. The uveal tract has three parts: the *iris*, which is the colored part of the eye and is the only part of the uvea we can see from the outside; the *ciliary body*, which makes fluid that bathes the lens and cornea and is also made up of muscles that help your eye focus; and the *choroid*, which contains blood vessels that feed all parts of the retina (see Figure 5.1).

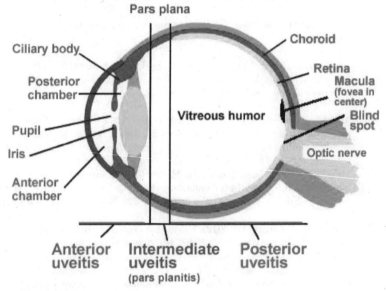

▲ Figure 5.1
Types of uveitis
Source: J. Zeis

Uveal tract problems include anterior uveitis (inflammation of the uveal tract in the front of the eye, including the iris; an inflamed iris is called iritis); intermediate uveitis, also called *pars planitis* (inflammation of the pars plana, part of the ciliary body); posterior uveitis (inflammation of the uveal tract in the back of the eye); and panuveitis (inflammation of the whole uveal tract, as well as the retina and vitreous—the clear gel in the middle of the eye).

According to the ISG Criteria (see Question 15), only certain types of eye problems can be used to help diagnose a case of Behçet's: anterior uveitis, posterior uveitis, inflammatory cells seen in the vitreous through a slit-lamp exam in an ophthalmologist's office, and/or retinal vasculitis (inflammation of retinal blood vessels).

An ophthalmologist uses a slit lamp to look at all parts of a patient's eyes to see if there is any inflammation or other problems. Watch an explanation of a dilated eye exam here: http://youtu.be/Yezth2mwffw?t=43s and watch a short slit-lamp exam here: http://youtu.be/p64u8BQUmbQ?t=3m13s

One out of every five Behçet's patients has eye inflammation (uveitis) as their first BD-related symptom, even before mouth ulcers. If you don't have any visual problems when your first Behçet's symptoms show up, you may get them within two to four years—keeping in mind that about one out of every four BD patients never gets eye disease. In addition, a 2014 study found that BD patients who get a lot of genital ulcers usually have less eye involvement.[10]

Besides the four types of eye involvement used to diagnose Behçet's, other eye problems have also been seen in BD patients: swelling of the retina, the macula (the main part of the retina where most of your vision focuses) and/or the optic disc (where all nerve cells leave the eye and form the optic nerve); orbital myositis[8] (pain when looking around, due to involvement of muscles that control eye movement); scleritis (inflammation of the sclera, the white outer covering of the eye); episcleritis (inflammation of an area of the sclera under the conjunctiva – the thin membrane that covers the inside of the eyelids and the sclera); choroiditis (inflammation of the blood vessel area between the sclera and retina); chorioretinitis (inflammation of the choroid and retina); optic papillitis (inflammation of the optic disc); and vitreous hemorrhage (bleeding into the vitreous). Other complications include the forming of cataracts, caused by constant inflammation and the use of corticosteroids; synechiae (when the colored part of the eye sticks to the cornea or lens, which keeps the pupil from moving); glaucoma; optic atrophy (wasting away of the optic nerve); papilledema (inflammation and swelling of the optic nerve); conjunctivitis; ulcers on the cornea; keratitis (corneal inflammation); ulcerations on the inside of the eyelids; retinal neovascularization (development of small, abnormal blood vessels in the retina); detached retina; optic neuropathy (damage to the optic nerve); epiretinal membrane (also called macular pucker, which is a layer of scar tissue that grows on the retinal surface, often on the macula where the fovea [the center of vision] is located); and hypopyon (pus in the front of the eye, which is rarely seen because many patients get treatment before this complication shows up).

23. If I have inflammation in one eye, will my other eye be affected too?

Not always. Many experts think it's guaranteed, but in a 2011 UK study,[1] 39 BD patients out of 107 with uveitis in one eye never developed problems in their other eye—even after five years of follow-up. Patients who did have involvement in the other eye usually had it within two years of their first-eye issues. Even if both of your eyes are affected, they may or may not be inflamed at the same time, and one eye may have less inflammation than the other.

24. What type of doctor should examine my eyes?

An ophthalmologist (an MD who specializes in the eyes) or a uveitis or retinal specialist is your best bet. Opticians and optometrists don't have the background or experience to diagnose and treat Behçet's-related eye disease. **Even if you've never had eye problems, every Behçet's patient should have a full eye/retinal exam with a specialist at least once a year.** That's because some BD eye problems can be "silent" at first, possibly damaging your retinas without causing any pain or changes in vision. Setting up a baseline exam and a long-term relationship with a uveitis specialist also gives you faster treatment options if you have questions or sudden, unexpected eye problems. If your eye problems are being caused by inflammation in your central nervous system, you may also need to see a neuro-ophthalmologist.

If you have Behçet's, it's important to pay attention to your eyes. Make an appointment right away if you have any of the following problems: eye pain; pain when looking at bright lights; redness around the iris (a "ciliary flush" —see Figure 5.2) or all through the white of the eye (see Figure 5.3); some loss of vision or change in any part of your vision; foggy vision that doesn't clear; a sudden increase in the number of floaters (stringy pieces of material that float around inside your eye, often seen when you look at the sky or a plain background); or flashes of light.

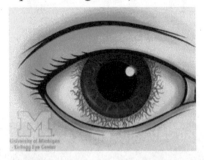

◀ **Figure 5.2**
Ciliary flush of iritis
Source: http://commons.wikimedia.org/
wiki/File:Ciliary-flush.jpg

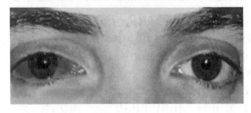

◀ **Figure 5.3**
Uveitis
Source: http://commons.
wikimedia.org/wiki/File:Iritis.jpg

Also, keep an Amsler Grid on hand (see Figure 5.4) and check your vision in each eye on a regular basis. Focus on the black dot in the center of the grid. If any of the lines on the grid seem wavy or don't look normal, or any pieces of the grid are missing, you may have retinal problems that need to be checked out. Call your ophthalmologist.

If you don't know whether your eye problem is serious, it's best to be careful: see an ophthalmologist or uveitis specialist. Don't wait, because some Behçet's-related eye problems can cause permanent damage or vision loss if they're not treated. If you don't have a regular ophthalmologist and need to see someone right away, try to find an eye hospital that has its own emergency room (for example, Massachusetts Eye and Ear Infirmary). If that's not possible and you have to call an ophthalmologist or uveitis specialist that you don't know, always say that you have Behçet's or a possible Behçet's diagnosis; you may be seen more quickly.

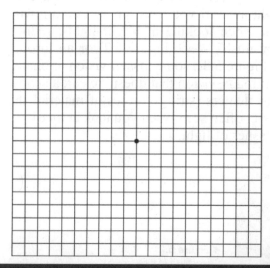

◄ Figure 5.4
Amsler Grid
Source:
http://commons.
wikimedia.org/wiki/
File:Normalamslergrid.gif

26. Is it okay to have eye surgery (like cataract removal or Lasik) if you have Behçet's?

That depends. Most experts believe cataract surgery and lens replacement in BD patients can be safe and successful, as long as the eye hasn't had any inflammation for at least three months before the operation. Anti-inflammatory medication like prednisone should be prescribed before and after surgery so there's less chance of complications.[2] Infliximab and interferon-alpha can also help lower the risk of eye problems with cataract and glaucoma surgery.[5,6]

Lasik surgery is a little different. Lasik is when a doctor uses a laser to change the shape of a person's cornea to improve vision and to (hopefully) get rid of the need for glasses or contacts. When the FDA first approved this type of surgery, they published a list of contraindications—diseases or conditions that might cause a problem for people having the operation. Eye diseases were on the list, along with autoimmune and connective-tissue diseases: there's a fear that Lasik surgery might cause eye inflammation in those patients, or scars on the cornea. There's also a chance Lasik could make a person's dry-eye problems much worse. Some studies of Lasik in autoimmune patients have shown good results, but more research is needed.[7]

27. Can I wear contact lenses if I have Behçet's?

Probably—but if you do, you might have some unexpected issues. A 2008 report[9] described a woman with BD who'd been wearing soft contact lenses successfully for 15 years, when her lenses suddenly stopped fitting. Tests done at an ophthalmologist's office showed that the centers of both of her corneas had started to flatten. In a process that kept going over several months, the shape of her corneas continued to change and her vision got worse. Her corneas went back to normal after 10 months of follow-up, when she was able to wear her original lenses again. While this is only a single case, the author has come across other Behçet's patients who've had the same problem with contacts that suddenly don't fit their eyes.

People who have dry eyes may also have problems wearing contacts.

28. Am I going to go blind?

As long as you get prompt treatment for any eye problems that show up, and they don't start with an **irreversible**, severe loss of vision (vision of 20/200 or worse that can't be corrected after six months of treatment), you have a good chance of keeping useful vision long term. That's because immunosuppressives, interferon alpha and newer anti-TNF treatments like infliximab—either alone or together—have a better track record of controlling BD-related eye inflammation than the treatments Behçet's patients were given in the 1980s and earlier. In fact, 50–90% of BD patients in Japan and Turkey and 25% of US BD patients became legally blind in the 1980s despite treatment. The chance of having severe visual loss has been cut in half since then, according to a 2011 UK[1] study.

The types of Behçet's-related eye problems that can lead to severe and permanent vision loss mostly affect blood vessels at the back of the eye. These vessels may get blocked or become narrow due to inflammation, which reduces or completely stops blood flow through parts of the retina. Once blood flow stops, the involved tissues die and vision is lost.

The risk of severe vision loss or blindness usually goes up every time a new symptom flare-up damages the retina. Here are some other risk factors linked to severe vision loss after 5 and 10 years of eye involvement:[1] men generally have a worse outcome than women, with more posterior uveitis, more vision loss and more severe loss of vision; people who only have inflammation in one eye have a worse long-term outcome than people who have both eyes involved (it may be due to ophthalmologists who are afraid to use high doses of immunosuppressive drugs when only one eye is affected); and treatment that doesn't include biologics like infliximab often leads to a worse outcome.

These days, most uveitis and retinal specialists don't take chances. They use prompt, aggressive treatments to stop any Behçet's-related eye inflammation, and to keep possible complications under control. See Chapter 13 for more information on treatments for eye disease and other issues.

REFERENCES

References

CHAPTER 5

1. Taylor, S. R., Singh, J., Menezo, V., Wakefield, D., McCluskey, P., & Lightman, S. (2011). Behçet disease: visual prognosis and factors influencing the development of visual loss. *American journal of ophthalmology, 152(6),* 1059–1066.

2. Ozyazgan, Y., & Bodaghi, B. (2010). Eye disease in Behçet's syndrome. In Yazici, H. & Yazici, Y. (Eds.), *Behçet's Syndrome* (pp. 73–94). New York, NY: Springer.

3. Zeis, J. (2003). *Essential Guide to Behçet's Disease.* Uxbridge, MA: Central Vision Press.

4. Kidd, D. P. (2013). Optic neuropathy in Behçet's syndrome. *Journal of neurology, 260(12),* 3065–3070.

5. Nishida, T., Shibuya, E., Asukata, Y., Nakamura, S., Ishihara, M., Hayashi, K., Takeno, M., Ishigatsubo, Y., & Mizuki, N. (2011). Clinical Course before and after Cataract and Glaucoma Surgery under Systemic Infliximab Therapy in Patients with Behçet's Disease. *Case reports in ophthalmology, 2(2),* 189–192. Available online at http://www.ncbi.nlm.nih.gov/pmc/articles/PMC3124456/

6. Krause, L., Altenburg, A., Bechrakis, N. E., Willerding, G., Zouboulis, C. C., & Foerster, M. H. (2007). Intraocular surgery under systemic interferon-alpha therapy in ocular Adamantiades-Behçet's disease. *Graefe's archive for clinical and experimental ophthalmology = Albrecht von Graefes Archiv für klinische und experimentelle Ophthalmologie, 245(11),* 1617–1621.

7. Mohammadpour, M. (2007). Excimer laser refractive surgery in patients with underlying autoimmune diseases. *Journal of cataract and refractive surgery, 33(2)*, 175; author reply 175–6.

8. Roh, J. H., Koh, S. B., & Kim, J. H. (2006). Orbital myositis in Behçet's disease: A case report with MRI findings. *European neurology, 56(1)*, 44–45.

9. Sañudo-Buitrago, F., González-Méijome, J. M., Bueno-Jimeno, I., Navarrete-Sanchís, J. N., & León-Jiménez, N. (2008). Topographic and refractive changes in a patient with contact lens intolerance associated with Behçet disease. *The British journal of ophthalmology, 92(3)*, 438–440.

10. Faezi, S. T., Chams-Davatchi, C., Ghodsi, S. Z., Shahram, F., Nadji, A., Akhlaghi, M., Moradi, K...& Davatchi, F. (2014). Genital aphthosis in Behçet's disease: Is it associated with less eye involvement? *Rheumatology international. Published online first, 12 April.*

Behçet's and the nervous system

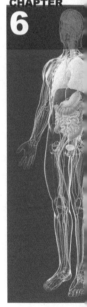

CHAPTER 6

For most people who have Behçet's, the possibility of developing neurological problems is scary and confusing. Some questions are common. For example, which medical problems can lead to a diagnosis of neuro-Behçet's (NBD)? Do headaches count? What symptoms should you watch out for? This chapter will try to take some of the mystery out of neurological complications and what they mean.

About one out of every five Behçet's patients develops neurological problems, but this number can be lower or higher depending on the country or region where you live (see Question 7). Very few people have neurological complications as their first symptom of Behçet's. If neurological problems appear at all, they usually show up after several years of other symptoms.

Keep the following in mind: neurological problems – like any health issues that people have – may be caused by medications you're taking or by other illnesses or issues **not** related to Behçet's or neuro-BD. For example, drugs like cyclosporin A, thalidomide, colchicine, and anti-TNF treatments may cause some side effects similar to symptoms found in neuro-Behçet's.

Don't make assumptions! Always see your doctor to ask questions and uncover the reasons for your specific symptoms.

29. Does Behçet's target the central nervous system or the peripheral nervous system? [1-5]

It can affect either one, but Behçet's-related neurological problems mostly affect the central nervous system (CNS). The CNS includes your brain and spinal cord. Involvement of the peripheral nervous system (PNS) can happen too, but less often. The PNS sends messages between the brain/spinal cord and your arms, legs, skin and organs. The PNS also controls the "automatic" functions of your body, like your heartbeat and ability to breathe (through the autonomic nervous system) and the voluntary movements of your body (through the somatic nervous system). See Question 32 to learn about signs and symptoms that Behçet's is affecting the peripheral nervous system.

There are two main types of neurological problems in Behçet's: problems caused by inflammation in or around the brain or spinal cord (parenchymal problems) and ones that are caused by aneurysms or by the development of blood clots in the brain (non-parenchymal problems).

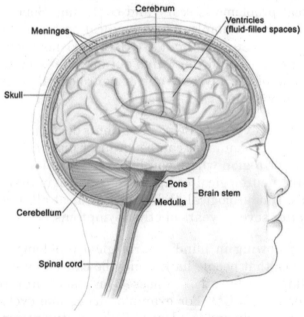

▲ Figure 6.1
Brain and brainstem
Source: http://seer.cancer.gov/statfacts/html/brain.html

30. What is parenchymal involvement in neuro-Behçet's?

Behçet's may cause inflammation in or around the brain, brainstem, or spinal cord in some people; this is called parenchymal involvement. It's not infectious—no one else can catch it from you. Symptoms depend on which part of the brain/spinal cord is affected and how badly it's inflamed. For example, meningoencephalitis—inflammation of the brain and the meninges, its protective covering—may start with a headache that gets worse over several days; infection and other possible causes would need to be ruled out first before considering Behçet's. See Figure 6.1 for an illustration of the brain and brainstem. **(Caution: not all headaches are serious! See Question 35.)**

People with meningoencephalitis may have a fever and a very stiff neck, feel sleepy, and/or have an increased sensitivity to pain or touch. If lesions develop in the brainstem—a favorite place for Behçet's inflammation—they may affect one or more of the cranial nerves located there. Cranial nerves start in the brain or brainstem and connect to nerves in the face, mouth, ears, eyes and throat. Cranial nerve problems may cause weakness in the facial muscles; double vision; constant, involuntary eyeball movements (*nystagmus*); a drooping eyelid; trouble swallowing; slurred speech or difficulty speaking; hearing loss; and/or dizziness or loss of balance.

Inflammation or lesions in other parts of the brain, brainstem, or spinal cord may cause numbness, loss of sensation, or weakness on one side of the body—similar to a stroke. Other possible problems include impotence (not being able to get or keep an erection); seizures (see Question 36); a loss of bladder or bowel control; a need to urinate often; or development of tremors, muscle contractions, and/or other movements you can't control. Some large lesions in the

Senses/abilities controlled by the 12 cranial nerves

I   Smell
II Optic nerve
III Eye movements: up/down/inward
IV Eye movements: downward/inward
V   Trigeminal nerve: facial sensation/movement
VI Lateral (sideways) eye movement
VII Facial movement
VIII Hearing and balance
IX Tongue and throat
X   Swallowing; muscles for voice
XI Neck and upper back movement
XII Tongue movement for swallowing/speech

brainstem and other parts of the brain may be mistaken for tumors.[4] Most of these cases have responded to corticosteroid treatment.

Doctors sometimes find optic neuropathy (damage to the optic nerve) and optic neuritis (inflammation/swelling of the optic nerve) in people with neuro-Behçet's, but these problems can also appear in people who don't have BD. Optic nerve issues may lead to "washed-out" color vision, pain when moving the eye, or loss of vision.

Some people with Behçet's have "silent" neurologic involvement. In other words, they don't have any obvious health complaints other than headaches and occasional fatigue or dizziness, but they've had abnormal results on neurological exams. For example, there may be abnormalities on MRI scans (brainstem, basal ganglia, or white matter lesions); on neuropsychological tests (mostly mild to moderate problems with attention, memory, and executive functions such as planning and problem-solving abilities); evoked potential studies (measuring how long it takes nerves to react when they're stimulated); and cerebrospinal fluid (CSF) analyses (mild pleocytosis, an abnormal increase in the number of cells in the CSF).[5] Experts are mixed on whether—or if—silent neuro involvement affects patients' long-term health. Regardless, brainstem lesions deserve extra investigation.

31. What is *non*-parenchymal involvement in neuro-Behçet's?

Blood clots or aneurysms in the brain are examples of non-parenchymal involvement.

Cerebral venous sinus thrombosis (CVT or CVST) is the presence of one or more blood clots (thromboses) in blood vessels that carry blood from the brain back to the heart. These clots may increase the cerebrospinal fluid (CSF) pressure in the brain. Cerebrospinal fluid surrounds the brain and spinal cord and acts like a protective cushion.

Signs of CVT include a headache that worsens over time or happens suddenly and severely; loss of vision, or abnormal vision due to *papilledema* (swelling of the optic disc); seizures; stroke-like symptoms; and/or mental confusion. Some patients may have a rise in CSF pressure in the brain that's not caused by a clot; this issue is called intracranial hypertension or pseudotumor cerebri, and it may cause symptoms similar to a CVT.

CVT is less common in adults than the neuro-BD problems caused by inflammation. However, children with neuro-Behçet's have the opposite problem—CVT is **more** common for them than brain or spinal cord inflammation (see Question 63).

Other possible non-parenchymal problems include:
- *Intracranial aneurysm*: When a weak spot in a blood vessel in the brain balloons out and fills with blood. This aneurysm may press on other parts of the brain, causing pain above or behind an eye; vision changes (including double vision); a pupil that gets large and stays that way; and/or stroke-like symptoms, like numbness or weakness on one side of the face or an eyelid that droops. An aneurysm that leaks or ruptures is a medical emergency. It can cause a sudden and very severe headache along with any of the following: nausea and vomiting, blurred/double vision, mental confusion, a seizure, stiff neck, light sensitivity, and/or loss of consciousness.
- *Cervical extracranial aneurysm/dissection*: A rupture, leak or tear of the carotid artery in the neck. It may lead to a stroke.
- *Acute meningeal syndrome.* Acute meningeal syndrome can cause headache, neck stiffness, fever, confusion, vomiting and/or trouble tolerating light or loud noises.

32. What are some other medical issues of neuro-Behçet's?

Peripheral nervous system involvement is supposedly rare in Behçet's, but includes:
- *Peripheral neuropathy* (damage to nerves that carry information from the spinal cord to other parts of the body, and vice versa) and *mononeuritis multiplex* (damage to at least two separate areas of peripheral nerves). Peripheral neuropathy can cause weakness, numbness, pins-and-needles sensations and/or tingling in the hands/arms or feet/legs, or a sharp, stabbing, or shock-like pain.
- *Myopathy* (muscle weakness) and *myositis* (inflammation of muscles).

- *Autonomic nervous system (ANS) involvement.*[6,7] The ANS controls mostly involuntary actions in the body, like heart rate, pupil size, digestion, sweating, and the widening/narrowing of blood vessels to help a person adjust to temperature extremes. When the ANS isn't working right, it can lead to erectile dysfunction, bladder problems, orthostatic hypotension (a sudden drop in blood pressure when standing up, which can cause dizziness, lightheadedness, a temporary decrease in hearing or vision, or fainting), heat intolerance, and postural orthostatic tachycardia syndrome (POTS). POTS causes a heart rate increase of 30 beats per minute or more—or over 120 total beats per minute—within the first 10 minutes of standing. POTS may cause heart palpitations, nausea, shaking, fainting, and lightheadedness. As a result, people with severe cases may have trouble handling even normal day-to-day activities.

  A 2009 report[16] also talks about "sympathetic storms" in a patient with neuro-BD. A sympathetic storm is an autonomic nervous system in overdrive. It can cause an abnormally high body temperature due to problems with the way the body handles heat (hyperthermia), high blood pressure, a faster than normal heart rate, and—sometimes—uncontrollable sweating.

33. Can Behçet's cause psychiatric or cognitive problems?

Yes. Some people with neuro-Behçet's may show changes in behavior that get worse with time and aren't linked to the use of corticosteroids or other medications. There may be episodes of any of the following: intense feelings of happiness and joy; doing things suddenly, without thinking of the result; mental confusion; not caring about social rules and guidelines; anxiety or nervous excitement; paranoia ("everyone is out to get me"); personality changes; dementia (not able to think well enough to do normal daily activities, solve problems, or control emotions); hallucinations; or performing actions that don't have a purpose, like pacing around a room or hand-wringing.[2,10] This "neuro-psycho-Behçet's syndrome" is often linked to a chronic progressive course of neuro-Behçet's[2]—in other words, it continues for a long time and keeps getting worse.

Possible mental changes in neuro-Behçet's patients include memory problems, especially loss of visuospatial long-term memory (remembering what objects looked like and how they were placed near each other) and short-term memory loss.[2,8] Even BD patients without obvious neurological problems or depression may have problems with executive functions; in other words, they may not be able to think clearly, make plans, set goals, and/or change their plans based on changed objectives.[9]

How do doctors test for neurological problems? Watch a full neurological exam performed on a patient (~25 minutes) at https://www.youtube.com/watch?v=V2MBiS1kc_0

ON THE WEB

34. How do specialists diagnose neuro-Behçet's? [For clinicians]

The 2013 International Consensus Recommendation for the Diagnosis and Management of Neuro-Behçet's Disease[1] (NBD) was created with the cooperation of 52 international experts in Behçet's disease, including 22 neurologists. These recommendations have helped de-mystify NBD diagnosis for many clinicians, although the proposed criteria still need to be validated in future studies.

For anyone unfamiliar with neuro-Behçet's and facing a possible NBD diagnosis in one of their patients, the full International Consensus Recommendation can be accessed online.[1] Highlights, however, are provided below.

The international group recommends a **definite** neuro-Behçet's diagnosis in the following type of patient:

- Meets the International Study Group criteria for BD (see Question 15)
- Has a recognized neurological syndrome (see Table 6.1) with neurological signs accepted as part of BD. It should be supported by either neuroimaging **or** CSF findings (see Table 6.2)
- Has no better explanation for the patient's neurological symptoms

The international group recommends a **probable** neuro-Behçet's diagnosis in the following type of patient, when there appears to be no better reason for the patient's neurological symptoms:

- Doesn't meet the full International Study Group criteria for BD (see Question 15), but has a neurological syndrome as described in Table 6.1, as well as some other BD-type signs/symptoms

OR

- Meets the International Study Group criteria for BD and has a *non*-characteristic neurological syndrome

Table 6.1 Neurological syndromes recognized by the International Consensus Recommendation

Parenchymal (one or more of the following):
• *Brainstem involvement*: Includes cerebellar or pyramidal dysfunction, cranial neuropathy, and ophthalmoparesis
• *Multifocal (diffuse) involvement*: Variable combination of brainstem signs and symptoms, cerebral or spinal cord involvement
• *Myelopathy*
• *Cerebral hemispheric involvement*: Includes encephalopathy, hemiparesis, hemisensory loss, seizures, dysphagia, and mental changes such as cognitive dysfunction or psychosis
• *Optic neuropathy*

Non-parenchymal
• Cerebral venous thrombosis
• Intracranial hypertension syndrome (pseudotumour cerebri)
• Acute meningeal syndrome

Table 6.2 Characteristic MRI and CSF findings in neuro-BD

MRI, parenchymal NBD
Location of lesions
• Brainstem is typical site: usually involves the pons, possibly extending up to involve the midbrain, basal ganglion and diencephalon
• In cerebral presentation: multiple small, white matter lesions; possible isolated cerebral hemisphere lesions need differential diagnosis from tumor, abscess, etc.
• Cervical or thoracic cord: single or multiple inflammatory lesions of variable length, often with brainstem, basal ganglia, or cerebral lesions seen at the same time. Isolated spinal cord lesions are rare

Types of lesions: Acute/subacute

- Hypo-intense to iso-intense on T1-weighted images, usually enhanced with contrast on Gad-T1W images
- Hyper-intense on T2W, FLAIR and diffusion-weighted images
- Restricted apparent diffusion coefficient on ADC map

Types of lesions: Chronic phase

- Possible smaller, non-enhancing lesions that may resolve on their own
- Nonspecific white matter lesions
- Possible atrophy, especially in the brainstem

MRI, non-parenchymal NBD

- Evidence of cerebral sinus or vein thrombosis on MR or CT venography
- Intracranial hypertension syndrome shows normal appearances
- Acute meningeal syndrome shows meningeal enhancement, especially on Gad-T1W images

Typical CSF findings

- Inflammatory changes that include increased cells, increased protein, and/or high IL-6.

35. If I have headaches, does that mean I have neuro-Behçet's?

Probably not. Headaches occur in about seven out of every ten Behçet's patients on a regular basis, but only **one** of those patients will have headaches that are directly caused by neurological involvement.[2,4] The most common types of BD-related headaches are migraine and tension-type headaches, which are similar to those in healthy people. These headaches may last for days.

Read the full 2013 *International Consensus Recommendation for* ON THE WEB *Diagnosis and Management of Neuro-Behçet's Disease* here: http://link.springer.com/content/pdf/10.1007%2Fs00415-013-7209-3.pdf .

Some headaches may be triggered by—or get worse with—BD symptom flare-ups. Active uveitis can also cause headaches.

The 10% of headaches due to neuro-Behçet's may be caused by inflammation in the brain (meningoencephalitis); inflammation of the lining of the brain (meningitis); or problems with increased CSF pressure in the brain due to cerebral venous sinus thrombosis (see Question 31).

BD patients with headaches should be checked further when their headaches are:[1]
- Getting worse over time
- Hard to control or persistent
- Severe enough that the person is unable to work, move or function normally
- Different from usual headaches, or the first and worst headache(s) ever
- Happening at the same time as neurological signs and symptoms

36. Can neuro-Behçet's cause seizures?

Yes. Types of seizures include tonic-clonic convulsions (also known as grand mal seizures, affecting the whole brain); partial seizures, including simple focal seizures where the person doesn't lose consciousness and stays aware of his surroundings; complex partial seizures, where the person may or may not remember the seizure itself; and myoclonic seizures, which are very fast jerks or twitches in a single muscle or group of muscles. These myoclonic jerks can happen to people in everyday life, too; on their own, they aren't evidence for a neuro-Behçet's diagnosis.

Depending on where a seizure begins in the brain, any of the following symptoms may occur: abnormal muscle contractions; staring spells with or without repetitive body movements; turning of the eyes that can't be controlled; abnormal sensations like numbness, tingling, or skin-crawling feelings; hallucinations; rapid heart rate/pulse; and dilated (big) pupils.

37. When are memory problems normal and when should I worry?

As we've seen in Question 32, some neuro-BD patients may have memory problems that get worse with time. However, memory problems can also happen in people who don't have Behçet's. We all occasionally lose car keys or forget why we've come into a room. So when is it *really* time to worry?

A serious memory problem can make it hard to do everyday things like driving, shopping, or even talking.[12] Speak with your doctor if you:

- Learn that you're asking the same questions over and over in a short period of time
- Aren't able to make or coordinate plans, or follow simple directions like in a recipe you've made many times before
- Get lost in places you know well
- Don't recognize people and places you've known for years
- Don't understand what you're seeing, or can't follow what people are saying to you
- Don't remember how to take care of yourself, like bathing, eating properly, shopping, or balancing a checkbook
- Don't remember how to dress yourself
- Withdraw from social activities

If you're experiencing memory loss, or friends/relatives are mentioning it to you, your doctor will probably run some tests. He or she will want to make sure your memory issues aren't being caused by an illness, a problem with your diet, depression, stroke, medication or other reason. Some medications that may affect memory[11] include: antianxiety drugs like diazepam (Valium) and lorazepam (Ativan); cholesterol-lowering drugs (statins) like atorvastatin (Lipitor) and simvastatin (Zocor); antiseizure drugs like gabapentin (Neurontin) and pregabalin (Lyrica); tricyclic antidepressants like amitriptyline (Elavil) and imipramine (Tofranil); narcotic painkillers like fentanyl (Duragesic) and oxycodone (OxyContin, Percocet); Parkinson's drugs (dopamine agonists) like apomorphine (Apokyn); hypertension drugs (beta-blockers) like propranolol (Inderal); sleeping aids like eszopicione (Lunesta) and zolpidem (Ambien); incontinence drugs for overactive bladder like oxybutynin (Oxytrol); and antihistamines like chlorpheniramine (Chlor-Trimeton) and diphenhydramine (Benadryl).

38. What can I expect long-term if I have neuro-Behçet's? [1,2,4,14,15]

Neuro-Behçet's disease (NBD) can be a hard diagnosis for patients to receive, but not all neuro-BD cases are the same in terms of complications and long-term effects. As a result, it's hard to make predictions for any individual case of NBD, including how well that person's neurological symptoms will react to different treatments.

Neuro-Behçet's is typically divided into three types of cases:

1. **Acute**: Approximately one out of every three neuro-BD patients has a single attack of neurological symptoms, with no other neuro involvement afterwards.[4]

2. **Relapsing**: Another one-third of neuro-BD patients have repeated attacks with a period of remission (no symptoms) between them.[4,14] Even though several studies have shown no link between a patient's HLA-B5 or HLA-B51 status and relapses of neurological symptoms, a 2014 study shows that at least half of neuro-BD patients relapse if they're HLA-B51 positive.[14]

3. **Progressive**: The final one-third of neuro-BD patients has a chronic progressive course, with impairments and/or disability that gets worse over time.[4]

In a 2009 report that tracked neuro-BD patients over ten years,[15] three out of four patients had at least a mild level of disability (EDSS ≥ 3) ten years after the start of their neurological problems. Almost half of the patients, though, showed moderate to severe levels of disability after ten years (EDSS ≥ 6). Researchers used the Expanded Disability Status Scale (EDSS) to measure disability: a "3" shows the ability to walk from place to place independently, with or without a cane, walker, or other aid; a person with a score of "6" needs at least one-sided assistance to walk for 100 meters (about the length of a football field), as well as assistance on activities of daily living, such as getting dressed and eating.

Factors that may lead to being disabled over the long term include:
- Weakness on one side of the body (*hemiparesis*) or partial paralysis of the lower limbs (*paraparesis*), and/or being severely disabled the first time neurological signs/symptoms show up
- Inflammatory lesions in the brainstem on MRI scans when neurological symptoms first appear
- Spinal cord lesions

- High pleocytosis and raised protein levels in cerebrospinal fluid (CSF)
- A progressive disease course that keeps getting worse
- Frequent neurological relapses, along with disabilities that don't go away even when symptoms have stopped
- Neurological relapses when tapering down to lower levels of steroids

Factors that may have a better long-term result include:
- "Silent" neurological involvement without any obvious symptoms
- Neurological symptoms that start with headache
- A single, acute neurological attack
- Central venous sinus thrombosis (CVT) and intracranial hypertension: if treated promptly and appropriately, it has a low risk of happening again

Remember, every patient is different, and no results are set in stone—even with neuro-BD.

References

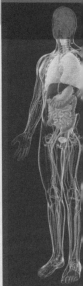

REFERENCES

CHAPTER 6

1. Kalra, S., Silman, A., Akman-Demir, G., Bohlega, S., Borhani-Haghighi, A., Constantinescu...Siva, A., & Al-Araji, A. (2013). Diagnosis and management of neuro-Behçet's disease: international consensus recommendations. *Journal of neurology, Published online 24 December 2013*. Available at http://link.springer.com/article/10.1007%2Fs00415-013-7209-3

2. Siva, A. & Hirohata, S. (2010). Behçet's syndrome and the nervous system. In Yazici, H. & Yazici, Y. (Eds.), *Behçet's Syndrome* (pp. 95-114). New York, NY: Springer.

3. Zeis, J. (2003). Neurological complications and neuro-BD. In *Essential Guide to Behçet's Disease* (pp. 125-136). Uxbridge, MA: Central Vision Press.

4. Al-Araji, A., & Kidd, D. P. (2009). Neuro-Behçet's disease: epidemiology, clinical characteristics, and management. *Lancet neurology, 8(2)*, 192–204.

5. Yesilot, N., Shehu, M., Oktem-Tanor, O., Serdaroglu, P., & Akman-Demir, G. (2006). Silent neurological involvement in Behçet's disease. *Clinical and experimental rheumatology, 5 Suppl 42*, S65-70. Available online at http://www.clinexprheumatol.org/pubmed/find-pii.asp?pii=17067430

6. Tellioglu, T., & Robertson, D. (2001). Orthostatic intolerance in Behcet's disease. *Autonomic neuroscience: basic & clinical, 89(1-2)*, 96–99.

7. Karataş, G. K., Onder, M., & Meray, J. (2002). Autonomic nervous system involvement in Behçet's disease. *Rheumatology international, 22(4)*, 155–159.

8. Monastero, R., Camarda, C., Pipia, C., Lopez, G., Camarda, L. K., Baiamonte, V., Ferrante, A., Triolo, G., & Camarda, R. (2004). Cognitive impairment in Behçet's disease patients without overt neurological involvement. *Journal of the neurological sciences, 220(1-2)*, 99–9104.

9. Erberk-Ozen, N., Birol, A., Boratav, C., & Kocak, M. (2006). Executive dysfunctions and depression in Behçet's disease without explicit neurological involvement. *Psychiatry and clinical neurosciences, 60(4)*, 465–472.

10. Joseph, F. G., & Scolding, N. J. (2007). Neuro-Behçet's disease in Caucasians: a study of 22 patients. *European journal of neurology: the official journal of the European Federation of Neurological Societies, 14(2)*, 174–180.

11. Neel, Jr., Dr. A. B. (2013). 10 Drugs That May Cause Memory Loss. *AARP.* Available online at http://www.aarp.org/health/brain-health/info-05-2013/drugs-that-may-cause-memory-loss.html

12. *NIH: National Institute on Aging.* (2014). Differences between mild forgetfulness and more serious memory problems. Available online at http://www.nia.nih.gov/alzheimers/publication/understanding-memory-loss/differences-between-mild-forgetfulness-and-more

13. Fountain, E. M., & Dhurandhar, A. (2014). Neuro-Behçet's Disease: An Unusual Cause of Headache. *Journal of general internal medicine. Published online* first, 19 February 2014.

14. Noel, N., Bernard, R., Wechsler, B., Resche-Rigon, M., Depaz, R., Boutin, D. L., Piette, J. C., Drier, A., Dormont, D., Cacoub, P., & Saadoun, D. (2014). Long-Term Outcome of Neuro-Behçet's Disease. *Arthritis and rheumatism. Published online first, 8 January 2014.*

15. Siva, A., & Saip, S. (2009). The spectrum of nervous system involvement in Behçet's syndrome and its differential diagnosis. *Journal of neurology, 256(4)*, 513–529.

16. Gono, T., Murata, M., Kawaguchi, Y., Wakasugi, D., Soejima, M., Yamanaka, H., & Hara, M. (2008). Successful treatment for sympathetic storms in a patient with neuro-Behçet's disease. *Clinical rheumatology, 28(3)*, 357–359."

Behçet's and the gastrointestinal (GI) system

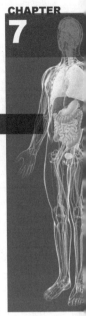

39. What parts of the GI tract can be affected by Behçet's?

Behçet's disease can affect any part of the gastrointestinal tract, from the mouth to the anus. Behçet's-related GI problems seem to happen most often in East Asian patients (usually from Japan and Korea), with a wide range of 0-40% of BD patients in other parts of the world.[1] *Intestinal Behçet's, entero-Behçet's* and *GI-Behçet's* are all terms used when gastrointestinal problems happen more often than Behçet's symptoms in other parts of the body.

Japanese researchers have come up with some guidelines for the diagnosis of intestinal Behçet's disease. Under the guidelines for intestinal Behçet's, patients must have:
- A characteristic oval-shaped, large ulcer in the terminal ileum

OR
- Inflammation or ulcerations in the large or small intestine

AND
- A diagnosis of Behçet's disease according to the ISG Classification Criteria (see Question 15)

Other parts of the GI tract and abdomen that may have BD involvement (Figure 7.1) include:
- *Cecum*: The pouch that connects the small and large intestines.
- *Colon*: The large intestine; it removes water and salt from digested matter and creates stool. Three main parts of the colon (the ascending colon, the transverse colon and the descending colon) can be seen in Figure 7.1.
- *Esophagus*: The tube that carries food, liquids and saliva from the mouth to the stomach.
- *Liver*: Among other functions, the liver makes bile to help digest lipids (fats). The gallbladder stores bile for use when it's needed.

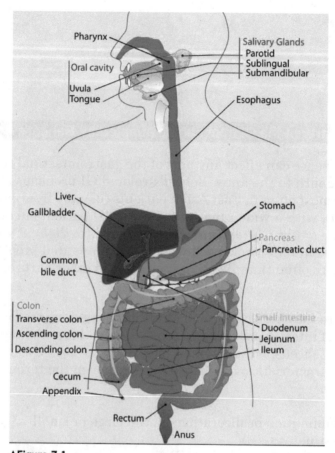

▲Figure 7.1
The gastrointestinal system
Source: http://commons.wikimedia.org/wiki/File:Digestive_system_diagram_en.svg

- *Pancreas*: Produces pancreatic juice with enzymes that help digest and absorb nutrients in the small intestine.
- *Spleen*: Helps to filter red blood cells and works as part of the immune system by making white blood cells to fight infection.
- *Small intestine*: Where most food digestion and absorption takes place. It has three parts:
  - The *duodenum*: the first part of the small intestine, located between the stomach and the jejunum
  - The *jejunum*: the middle part of the small intestine
  - The *ileum*: the final and longest part of the small intestine. The *terminal ileum* is the end of the small intestine where it connects to the cecum.

Here are some more definitions that can help when talking about GI-BD:

- *Erosions*: Erosions are caused by inflammation, wearing away and/or ulceration of the membrane lining the stomach
- *Fistula*: An abnormal connection or passageway between two organs or vessels in the body. Plural is *fistulae*
- *Perforation*: A hole in the wall of a body part, like the small intestine or large intestine
- *Stricture*: Abnormal narrowing of a body passage, often caused by scar tissue
- *Varices*: Abnormally enlarged veins, with many "tortuous" twists and turns

Table 7.1 provides information on places other than the mouth where BD-related GI lesions and inflammation can happen.[2]

Table 7.1 Location of non-oral, Behçet's-related lesions

Location	Types of involvement
Esophagus	Aphthous ulcers, fistulae, esophageal varices, strictures, pseudomembranous esophagitis
Stomach	(Rare), aphthous ulcers, erosions
Duodenum	Aphthous ulcers, gastric emptying abnormalities (gastroparesis)
Terminal ileum/cecum and surrounding area	Aphthous ulcers
Colon	Aphthous, deep ("volcano-type") and/or oval ulcers (or rare longitudinal ulcers); mucosal inflammation
Rectum/anus	(Rare), inflammation, ulcers, fistulae, abscesses

(Contd.)

Location	Types of involvement
Liver	Fatty liver; cirrhosis; Budd-Chiari syndrome: hepatic vein and/or IVC (inferior vena cava) blockage causing abdominal pain, an enlarged liver, and accumulation of fluid in the abdomen; bile duct inflammation
Gallbladder	Problems with motility (ability of muscle contractions in the gallbladder to properly release the right amount of bile during digestion)[3]; possible low-grade inflammation of the lining of the gallbladder.
Spleen	Enlarged/inflamed spleen
Pancreas	(Rare), inflammation of the pancreas (pancreatitis)
Peritoneum	Inflammation of the peritoneum (peritonitis), the thin tissue that lines the inner wall of the abdomen and covers most of the abdominal organs.

Behçet's-related GI involvement can range from mild to severe. Severe involvement can lead to serious complications, such as deep ulcers, perforations and gastrointestinal bleeding. These problems may need long-term medical care, including surgery and follow-up. Factors that can affect outcomes in GI-BD patients include intestinal ulcers that are deep and volcano-shaped, intestinal perforation(s), a history of having corticosteroid treatment after surgery, high CRP levels, and positive ASCA (anti-saccharomyces cerevisiae antibodies).[9]

Read more about "Outcome predictors for intestinal Behçet's disease" in this 2013 article by Park, Kim, and Cheon: http://www.eymj.org/Synapse/Data/PDFData/0069YMJ/ymj-54-1084.pdf

ON THE WEB

The places where GI-Behçet's lesions show up most often are the terminal ileum and the cecum (the ileocecal region), followed by the ascending colon and the transverse colon.[4] Most patients with intestinal BD who have never had surgery of the colon (96%) have lesions in or near the ileum/cecum; 67% of those patients have only one ulcer.[9] While the other parts of the GI system listed in Table 7.1 may not have as much involvement, lesions can still happen in those places and may cause symptoms.

40. What types of GI symptoms can Behçet's patients have?

The most common symptoms of intestinal Behçet's are abdominal pain and/or tenderness, nausea, vomiting, changes in bowel habits (constipation, or diarrhea that may or may not include mucous and blood), gastrointestinal bleeding, and/or loss of weight. Symptoms often depend on where the lesions are located or on other problems in the GI tract. For example, ulcers in the esophagus may cause pain below the breastbone and trouble with swallowing. More serious complications in the esophagus are rare but still possible, such as bleeding, perforations, and fistulae. Crampy pain in the lower right abdomen could point to ulcers in the ileocecal area.

Deep intestinal ulcers, especially if they're perforated, may cause bleeding and will often need surgery (see Question 41).

Gastroparesis is rarely talked about in medical journals in connection with Behçet's, but the author has heard from many BD patients diagnosed with this problem. Gastroparesis is weakness of the stomach muscles and/or a problem with the nerves that control the stomach muscles. It causes delayed emptying of the stomach after eating. Gastroparesis can lead to pain in the upper and/or lower abdomen, nausea/vomiting, discomfort and a too-early feeling of fullness during meals, along with bloating and heartburn.[5] While gastroparesis may be caused by BD, opioid and narcotic medications can also slow down the speed of digestion. Other medications that can have an impact on gastric emptying include some antidepressants and anti-emetics, which are drugs to control nausea and motion sickness. In the case of a woman with BD and severe gastroparesis, her physicians successfully used a combination of infliximab (300 mg every eight weeks), methotrexate (20 mg SQ weekly) and dapsone (75 mg daily) to bring her digestion back to normal within four months.[6]

Some Behçet's patients have also been able to control their GI tract issues, such as diarrhea, abdominal pain, constipation, and weight loss, through the gluten-free diet normally followed by people with celiac disease. While there's no agreement about any link between Behçet's and celiac, some experts suggest doing blood tests and a small-bowel biopsy to rule out celiac in any BD patient with diarrhea who also has the "silent" celiac symptoms of anemia and iron deficiency.[7,8]

41. Can surgery in the GI tract be a problem for Behçet's patients?

Yes, for some patients. GI-Behçet's patients sometimes need surgery to remove a part of the intestines if they have serious complications like a hole in the intestines (perforation), or bleeding that doesn't stop. Unfortunately, in about half of these patients, new ulcers, deep lesions or fistulae may form in the intestines within two years of surgery. The actual surgical site—where bowel has been removed and the ends re-attached—may also have a pathergy-type reaction. Up to four out of five patients who've had repeat intestinal surgeries eventually have new lesions form at the site. These lesions can be hard to heal, and contents from the intestines may leak into the body. Experts recommend following these cases closely during the first two years after surgery.[1,2]

42. How can specialists tell the difference between Behçet's and Crohn's disease?

Even GI specialists can have trouble telling the difference between a person with intestinal Behçet's and one who has Crohn's or another inflammatory bowel disease, such as ulcerative colitis. Adding to the confusion, some patients can be diagnosed with both GI-Behçet's and Crohn's or another bowel disease at the same time. Table 7.2 lists some of the main differences between intestinal BD and Crohn's disease.

Table 7.2 Most common features of intestinal Behçet's disease vs Crohn's disease [1,2,4,9]

Feature	Intestinal BD	Crohn's disease
Ulcer shape:		
Round/oval and/or deep ("volcano")	Most common	Rare
Linear/longitudinal	Rare	Most common
Irregular/geographic [a]	Sometimes	Most common

Feature	Intestinal BD	Crohn's disease
Where ulcers form (distribution)		
Focal: Single or multiple (often with ≤ 6 ulcers)	Most common, especially in ileocecal region	Sometimes
Segmental ("skip lesions")	Sometimes	Most common
Diffuse	Sometimes	More common
Cobblestone appearance	Rare to none	Most common
Granulomas	Rare	Most common
HLA (not required for diagnosis):		
B51 and/or A26	More common	Rare
DR4 and/or DQ4	Rare	More common
Perianal disease	Rare	More common
Bowel perforation	Very common	Rare

[a] Shallow ulcers of various shapes, with distinct edges

Read about and see 34 radiological images of GI-BD findings in the colon:
ON THE WEB http://pubs.rsna.org/doi/pdf/10.1148/radiographics.21.4.g01jl19911
From *Radiologic findings of Behçet syndrome involving the gastrointestinal tract* (2001).

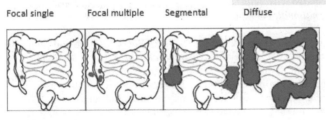

	Focal single	Focal multiple	Segmental	Diffuse
GI-BD[a]	63% (72/115)	35% (40/115)	2% (2/115)	1% (1/115)
Crohn's[b]	5% (7/135)	19% (26/135)	56% (75/135)	20% (27/135)

[a] n=115 [b] n=135

▲Figure 7.2
Comparison of lesion distribution patterns in 115 GI-Behcet's patients vs 135 Crohn's disease patients[4]
Source: Suggested by "Distribution pattern of lesions in GIBD"[1]

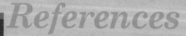

CHAPTER 7

1. Cheon, J. H., Celik, A. F., & Kim, W. H. (2010). Behçet's disease: Gastrointestinal involvement. In Yazici, H. & Yazici, Y. (Eds.), *Behçet's Syndrome.* (pp. 165-188). New York, NY: Springer.

2. Bayraktar, Y., Ozaslan, E., & Van Thiel, D. H. (2000). Gastrointestinal manifestations of Behçet's disease. *Journal of clinical gastroenterology, 30(2),* 144–154.

3. Yakut, M., Ustun, Y., Kabacam, G., Bektas, M., & Soykan, I. (2012). Gallbladder volume and ejection fraction in patients with Behçet's disease. *Clinics and research in hepatology and gastroenterology, 36(1),* 20-21.

4. Lee, S. K., Kim, B. K., Kim, T. I., & Kim, W. H. (2009). Differential diagnosis of intestinal Behçet's disease and Crohn's disease by colonoscopic findings. *Endoscopy, 41(1),* 9–16.

5. Bielefeldt, K. (2012). Gastroparesis: concepts, controversies, and challenges. *Scientifica, 2012, Article ID 424802. doi: 10.6064/2012/424802.* Available online at http://www.ncbi.nlm.nih.gov/pmc/articles/PMC3820446/

6. Fresno, R. B. (2002). Behcet disease associated with severe gastroparesis: A dramatic response to combination therapy with methotrexate and infliximab. *Arthritis & Rheumatism, 44*(S9), S120.

7. Caldas, C. A., Lage, L. V., & de Carvalho, J. F. (2010). Behçet's disease associated with celiac disease: a very rare association. *Rheumatology international, 30(4),* 523–525.

8. Ergul, B., Kocak, E., & Koklu, S. (2012). Behcet disease and celiac disease: to screen or not? *Rheumatology international, 32(8),* 2591–2592.

9. Grigg, E. L., Kane, S., & Katz, S. (2012). Mimicry and deception in inflammatory bowel disease and intestinal Behcet disease. *Gastroenterology & hepatology, 8(2),* 103–112. Available online at http://www.ncbi.nlm.nih.gov/pmc/articles/PMC3317507/

Behçet's and the ears, nose, and throat

43. Can Behçet's affect your hearing?[1,2]

Yes—but if it happens, it's often a mild or moderate amount of hearing loss in some of the higher frequencies, not necessarily in the lower frequencies of speech. As a result, you might have a problem and not know it, especially if you're still able to hear what people are saying to you. A 2013 study found there was a significant difference in hearing ability between BD patients and healthy people at the following frequencies: 1,000, 2,000, 4,000, and 8,000 Hz.[1] Any hearing loss may be in one ear only, or it may affect both ears at different frequencies.

Some studies have uncovered hearing loss in as many as four out of five people with Behçet's. The amount of hearing loss wasn't linked to their other BD-related symptoms or the length of time since they'd been diagnosed. However, older BD patients and those who've tested positive for HLA-B51 may have a greater chance of developing hearing problems.

Experts feel lesions or inflammation in the cochlea of the inner ear (see Figure 8.1) may be the cause of most Behçet's-related hearing loss. Doctors can't see this type of problem by looking in your ears with a light. An ENT (ear/nose/throat) professional has to do special testing on your ears to uncover the problem.

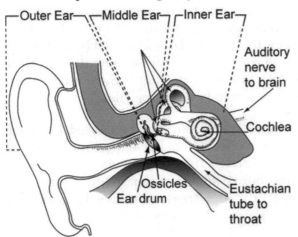

◄ **Figure 8.1**
The outer, middle and inner ear
Source: http://commons.wikimedia.org/
wiki/File:Outer,_middle_and_inner_ear.jpg

44. If you suddenly lose your hearing, can you get it back?

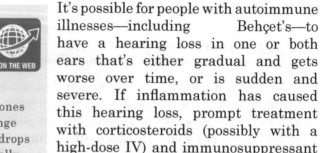

How's your hearing? Take the Online Tone Generator 60-second hearing test at http://onlinetonegenerator.com/hearingtest.html. Use headphones and sit through the **whole** range of tones, even if your hearing drops out at times. Researchers usually test BD patients at tones ranging from 250 to 8,000 Hz. See your doctor for more reliable testing if you notice any hearing loss during this online test.

It's possible for people with autoimmune illnesses—including Behçet's—to have a hearing loss in one or both ears that's either gradual and gets worse over time, or is sudden and severe. If inflammation has caused this hearing loss, prompt treatment with corticosteroids (possibly with a high-dose IV) and immunosuppressant drugs may completely return the hearing of some of these patients back to normal.[1,2,3]

A cochlear implant is an option for some BD patients who have a permanent hearing loss. These surgeries seem to go well, without the types of pathergy reactions that can happen in some GI-BD and other Behçet's-related operations. See Question 76 for more information about surgical outcomes in BD patients.

45. What happens if your inner ear is affected by Behçet's?[2,4,5]

The inner ear doesn't just help with hearing. It's also part of the *vestibular system*, which helps with balance and with your ability to keep objects in focus when your head is moving. People who have Behçet's-related inner-ear problems may report dizziness or vertigo, the feeling that the room is spinning around them. They may also hear the constant ringing, buzzing, hissing or clicking sounds of tinnitus, although tinnitus can also affect one out of every five healthy people. BD patients with inner-ear involvement might have constant eyeball movements that they can't control (nystagmus), or objects in front of them might seem to move back and forth at a steady speed (oscillate).

Any of the problems listed above can also be caused by other health problems besides Behçet's, so it's important to see a specialist. In particular, vertigo that occurs when lying down may actually be benign paroxysmal positional vertigo (BPPV). More information on BPPV and treatments can be found on Mayo Clinic's Website at http://www.mayoclinic.org/diseases-conditions/vertigo/basics/causes/con-20028216.

Some specific tests that can point to inner-ear damage include:

- The *caloric stimulation test*, where very cold or warm water is placed in the outer ear canal at different times. The doctor will look for specific eye movements during the test. This test is part of a full ENG/VNG (electronystagmography and videonystagmography) group of eye-movement tests.
- The *rotational chair test*, which helps record eye movements while the head moves at different speeds.

Learn more about tests of the vestibular system at the Vestibular Disorders Association Website: http://vestibular.org/understanding-vestibular-disorder/diagnosis

46. Can Behcet's cause ulcerations or lesions in your nose, or affect your sense of smell?

Yes. One of the largest studies of nasal involvement in Behçet's patients took place in 2010.[6] Sixty-seven BD patients out of 400 (17%) either had nasal issues at the time of the exam or a history of nasal problems, but nothing obvious on the day of the study. When doctors looked in the noses of the patients who had symptoms on the day of their appointment, 16 patients had issues that could be seen. Problems included nasal cartilage deformity, a one-sided nasal "obstruction" (not defined), non-aphthous ulcers, crusted ulcers, and/or post-nasal drip. The most commonly reported symptom was a distorted sense of smell, which occurred in half of the patients with current nasal problems.

A 2014 study looked at a much smaller group of 30 BD patients.[7] In this group, half of the patients had lesions inside their nose. The most common place for lesions and ulcerations was just inside the nostrils. The next most-common place was farther up inside the nose (the inferior turbinate) and the nasal septum (which divides the inside of the nose in two). One out of every three patients who have nasal lesions experience more pain and nosebleeds than those who don't have obvious lesions. Many of these lesions bleed easily.

This study also tested for any problems with the patients' sense of smell by using the CCCRC Olfactory Assessment. The CCCRC gives people "sniff tests" of common household items such as peanut butter, mothballs, coffee, and Vicks VapoRub. Out of the 30 BD patients in the study, eight had a slight problem with their ability to smell and detect odors, five had a moderate problem with their sense of smell, and five had a severe problem. However, none of these 18 patients felt they had *any* odor-detecting problems. Researchers aren't sure if these problems are caused by neurological issues or whether they're due to lesions, ulcers and other nasal troubles.

Some personal Behçet's contacts have also reported phantom smells (of burnt toast, for example) that no one else can notice. These odors may last for a few seconds or minutes. There's no evidence that phantom smells are directly related to BD, but they may be due to migraine auras, seizure activity, or other medical problems. See your doctor for more information.

47. Can Behcet's cause swelling or ulcerations in the throat?[8]

Yes. Behcet's-related ulcers or inflammation in the back of the throat may cause trouble with swallowing (dysphagia) or lead to a severe sore throat (pharyngitis) that's often mistaken for tonsillitis. The uvula, the small fleshy "punching bag" at the back of the throat, is a favorite location for ulcers and swelling. BD research studies have also found patients with ulcers on their tonsils, in the larynx (the voice box), the esophagus (the tube carrying food to the stomach), and the epiglottis (which keeps food from going into your windpipe). Figure 8.2 shows the parts of the throat.

People who have a lot of BD-related sore throats, ulcers in the esophagus, or GERD (gastroesophageal reflux disease) may

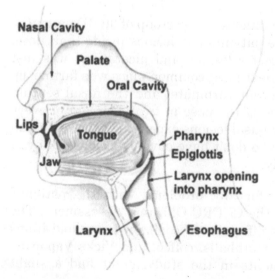

◄ **Figure 8.2**
Parts of the mouth and throat
Source: http://en.wikipedia.org/
wiki/File:Illu01_head_neck.jpg

sometimes develop scar tissue in the throat. Scarring may lead to stenosis (stricture)—a narrowing of the passageway. Stenosis can cause problems with swallowing. Doctors use an endoscopy or a barium swallow test to diagnose a stricture, which can then be treated with stretching (dilation) of the esophagus.

References

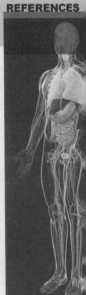

REFERENCES

CHAPTER 8

1. Kemal, O., Anadolu, Y., Boyvat, A., & Tataragasi, A. (2013). Behçet disease as a cause of hearing loss: A prospective, placebo-controlled study of 29 patients. *Ear, nose, & throat journal, 92(3)*, 112–120.

2. Calamia, K. T., & Fresko, I. (2010). Miscellaneous manifestations of Behçet's disease. In Yazici, H. & Yazici, Y. (Eds.), *Behçet's Syndrome*. (pp. 191–193). New York, NY: Springer.

3. Cinar, S., Cinar, F., & Kiran, S. (2012). Is there a need for audiologic evaluation in patients with Behçet disease? *Ear, nose, & throat journal, 91(3)*, E15-9.

4. Kulahli, I., Balci, K., Koseoglu, E., Yuce, I., Cagli, S., & Senturk, M. (2005). Audio-vestibular disturbances in Behcet's patients: report of 62 cases. *Hearing research, 1-2*, 28–31.

5. White, A. S., Taylor, R. L., McNeill, C., Garsia, R., & Welgampola, M. S. (2014). Behçet's disease presenting as a peripheral vestibulopathy. *Journal of clinical neuroscience: official journal of the Neurosurgical Society of Australasia. In press:* http://dx.doi.org/10.1016/j.jocn.2013.08.021

6. Shahram, F., Zarandy, M. M., Ibrahim, A., Ziaie, N., Saidi, M., Nabaei, B., & Davatchi, F. (2010). Nasal mucosal involvement in Behçet disease: a study of its incidence and characteristics in 400 patients. *Ear, nose, & throat journal, 89(1)*, 30–33.

7. Veyseller, B., Dogan, R., Ozucer, B., Aksoy, F., Meric, A., Su, O., & Ozturan, O. (2014). Olfactory function and nasal manifestations of Behçet's disease. *Auris, nasus, larynx, 41(2)*, 185–189.

8. Morales-Angulo, C., Vergara Pastrana, S., Obeso-Aguera, S., Acle, L., & Gonzalez-Gay, M. A. (2014). [Otorhinolaryngological manifestations in patients with Behçet disease]. *Acta otorrinolaringologica espanola, 65(1)*, 15–21. Available online in English at: http://zl.elsevier.es/en/revista/acta-otorrinolaringologica-espanola-402/pdf/90277880/S300/

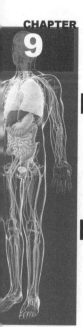

Behçet's and the cardiovascular system

48. What is the cardiovascular system?

The cardiovascular system (also called the circulatory system) is made up of the heart and all the veins, arteries and smaller blood vessels that carry blood through the body. When Behçet's directly affects blood vessels more often than other parts of the body, it's called vasculo-Behçet's.

49. Can Behçet's affect the heart?

Yes. A 2012 study of 807 Behçet's patients found 48 patients (6%) with heart involvement. Table 9.1 gives information on the serious types of heart complications that some BD patients may have.

Table 9.1 Heart problems found in some Behçet's disease patients [1,2,3,4]

Heart problem	What it means
Pericarditis	Inflammation of the pericardium— the sac that surrounds the heart. Pericarditis is the most common Behçet's-related heart problem.
Pericardial effusion	A buildup of fluid around the heart, in the pericardium.
Pericardial tamponade	Pressure on the heart, caused by fluid in the pericardium.
Constrictive pericarditis	The pericardium around the heart becomes thick and rigid from long-term inflammation, making it hard for the heart to stretch/beat properly and fill with blood.
Acute myocardial infarction	Heart attack. In young BD patients, it's usually due to coronary artery vasculitis (aneurysms or partial/total blockage of blood flow in coronary arteries).

Heart problem	What it means
Silent myocardial infarction	Heart attack with no chest pain or other symptoms.
Angina	Chest pain or discomfort when part of the heart muscle isn't getting enough oxygen-rich blood.
Intracardiac thrombus	Blood clot on the inside wall of a chamber of the heart. In BD patients, it occurs most often on the heart's right side, but has also been seen on the left. May extend to the vena cava and be linked with a pulmonary artery aneurysm (see Question 56).
Mitral or aortic valve prolapse	When the heart's mitral or aortic valve is "floppy" and doesn't close with a tight seal. May cause mitral or aortic insufficiency—the backflow of blood into a chamber of the heart.
Endocarditis	Inflammation of the endocardium, the inside lining of the heart's chambers and valves.
Myocarditis	Inflammation of the heart muscle.
Ventricular arrhythmias	Abnormal heart rhythms that start in the ventricles (the bottom chambers of the heart). Tachycardia (abnormally fast heart rhythm) is most common.
Congestive cardiomyopathy	When the heart becomes weak, enlarged and unable to pump blood normally.
Diastolic dysfunction	When one of the heart's ventricles is not filling properly with blood. The left ventricle is most often affected in BD patients.

(Contd.)

Heart problem	What it means
Aneurysm	When an artery wall is weakened and the diameter of the artery increases by at least 50%, creating a blood-filled bulge. This bulge is held in place by all three layers of the wall of the artery. It can either look like a balloon sticking out of a weak area of the artery, or it can increase the width of the whole artery in that area.
Pseudoaneurysm	Also called a false aneurysm, when leaking or pooling of blood outside a damaged blood vessel is held in place by surrounding tissue. May be caused by trauma that punctures the artery, or surgical procedures to access the blood vessel (like angiography). A mass that pulsates may have a pseudoaneurysm underneath it.
Electrical conduction problems	Electrical conduction stimulates the heart muscle to pump blood properly through the body. **For clinicians:** BD-related electrical problems include A-V block with presyncope, or syncope requiring a pacemaker; right bundle branch block; ventricular premature beats and ventricular tachycardia.

50. What symptoms might point to heart involvement?

Call your health care provider as soon as possible if you're worried about the way you feel and/or have any of the following symptoms:

- Chest discomfort or pain
- Chest pain when exercising
- Fainting
- Dizziness
- Shortness of breath or trouble breathing

- Heart palpitations (a racing/pounding heart or irregular heartbeat, whether you're active or resting)
- Coughing up blood

51. How do specialists check for heart involvement?

Specialists use a few different tests to check for heart involvement:
- Electrocardiogram (also called an EKG or ECG, which checks heart rhythms)
- Echocardiogram (uses ultrasound to make a moving picture of the heart)
- Doppler imaging (uses ultrasound to check how well blood is flowing in blood vessels)
- Holter monitor (a portable device you can wear that tracks your heart activity for at least 24 hours)
- Chest X-ray, CT scan, and/or MRI

52. What types of blood vessel problems can be caused by Behçet's?

Behçet's is a vascular illness that can inflame blood vessels of any size in the body. In general, men have more vascular problems than women. In one of the largest studies of blood vessel lesions in Behçet's patients[5], 332 patients out of 2319 (14%) had vascular involvement.

The veins of BD patients are affected more often than the arteries (85% vs. 15%). Veins carry blood back to the heart, while nearly all arteries (except the pulmonary artery) carry oxygen-rich blood from the heart to the rest of the body.

Inflammation in the blood vessels of Behçet's patients can sometimes cause the following complications (see Figure 9.1):
- *Thrombosis*: When a clot forms inside a blood vessel and keeps blood from flowing freely through the vessel.
- *Aneurysm*: When a weakness in the wall of a blood vessel causes a blood-filled bulge to form in the vessel wall.
- *Stenosis*: When the inside wall of a blood vessel gets thicker so the vessel itself gets narrower, less blood is able to flow through the opening.
- *Dissection* or *rupture*: A dissection is a tear in the wall of a blood vessel. It allows blood to flow between the layers of the vessel wall and separate them. A rupture is when a blood vessel bursts. This complication can be deadly.

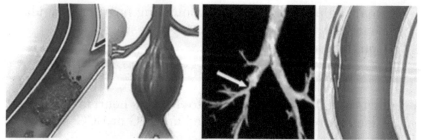

▲ Figure 9.1
Thrombosis (blood clot), aneurysm, stenosis, dissection
Source: J. Zeis composite from Wikipedia and Wikimedia Commons

53. What are the major vein-related problems for BD patients? [3,5,6]

- *Deep vein thrombosis (DVT)* is a blood clot in one of the deep veins under the skin, often in the legs. DVT is the most common type of vascular problem for Behçet's patients. It can cause swelling in the leg, including the foot and ankle; crampy pain in the calf and/or feet and ankles; and a feeling of warmth in the painful area. It may also cause an ulcer on the surface of the skin that has trouble healing. Common places where DVTs happen include the femoral and popliteal veins, inferior and superior vena cava, cerebral venous sinus, and iliac and hepatic veins. Since deep vein thromboses in BD seem to be caused by the inflammation of vessels instead of by blood-coagulation problems, some experts suggest treating them with immunosuppressants instead of (or along with) anticoagulants. Whether or not to use anticoagulation in Behçet's patients is an issue for many BD experts.
- *Claudication* can happen in up to one-third of BD patients with major vein involvement.[8] Claudication is limping, pain and/or difficulty in walking due to poor blood circulation in the affected area (often the calves or thighs).
- *Superficial thrombophlebitis* is also common. It can happen anywhere that a vein has been injured, often where an IV has been inserted in a vein just below the skin. Some BD experts think of superficial thrombophlebitis as a pathergy "substitute." It can cause pain when pressure is applied to the affected area. It can

also cause redness and inflammation and often results in a hardening of the vein.

- *Budd-Chiari syndrome* (BCS) is a rare but sometimes deadly complication of Behçet's. It's caused by blockage of the hepatic veins that drain the liver, and it's often linked to a blockage of the inferior vena cava (IVC) at the same time. The IVC carries blood from the lower part of the body directly into the heart. Signs and symptoms of BCS include severe upper abdominal pain, jaundice, an enlarged liver, elevated liver enzymes, and a swollen abdomen due to fluid buildup.

54. What are the major artery-related problems for BD patients?

Lesions in the arteries of BD patients aren't as common as lesions in the veins, but they're often more serious. Men with Behçet's develop problems in the arteries much more often than women, and these arterial lesions usually happen at the same time as venous thrombosis (blood clots in the veins). A 20-year study of 101 Behçet's patients with arterial involvement was published in 2012; it shows the following important results:[7]

- *Possible symptoms at the start of arterial involvement (most to least common)*: Abdominal pain, unexplained fever, hemoptysis (coughing up blood or blood-tinged sputum), chest pain, claudication (limping, pain or discomfort when walking), arterial ulcers, and weight loss.
- *Don't ignore unexplained fevers*: Unexplained fevers are more common in patients with aneurysms. The researchers recommend screening any BD patients for "silent" arterial lesions if they have unexplained fevers, phlebitis and/or an inflammatory syndrome.
- *Types of arterial problems (most to least common)*: Aneurysms, occlusions (blocked arteries), stenosis (narrowed artery), and aortitis (inflammation of the wall of the aorta).
- *Locations of arterial lesions (most to least common)*: Femoral, pulmonary, iliac, abdominal aorta, popliteal, tibial, thoracic aorta, heart, upper limb, cerebral, celiac trunk, renal, and mesenteric arteries. Lower limb lesions are much more common than upper limb.

- *The most common reason for an arterial lesion to form is trauma (injury) to the artery.* Types of trauma listed in this study include surgery, arteriography (a test where a special fluid is injected into the blood vessel to make it show up more clearly on pictures), arterial blood gas, and lung biopsy. **For clinicians:** The researchers recommend noninvasive imaging techniques to investigate arterial lesions since aneurysms have sometimes formed after arterial punctures, surgery or angiography in other studies. Immunosuppressants should also be used before surgery to reduce the chance of postoperative complications.
- *Most serious/deadly arterial lesions*: Thoracic and pulmonary arteries often have the most severe lesions. Pulmonary artery aneurysms (PAA) are the leading cause of death in Behçet's.[3]
- *Immunosuppressants can help*: BD patients in this study of arterial lesions had a much better long-term outcome when treated with immunosuppressants.

REFERENCES

References

CHAPTER 9

1. Sezen, Y., Buyukhatipoglu, H., Buyukatipoglu, H., Kucukdurmaz, Z., & Geyik, R. (2010). Cardiovascular involvement in Behçet's disease. *Clinical rheumatology, 29(1)*, 7–12.

2. Geri, G., Wechsler, B., Thi Huong, D. L., Isnard, R., Piette, J. C., Amoura, Z., Resche-Rigon, M., Cacoub, P., & Saadoun, D. (2012). Spectrum of cardiac lesions in Behçet disease: a series of 52 patients and review of the literature. *Medicine, 91(1)*, 25–34.

3. Hamuryudan, V., & Melikoglu, M. (2010). Vascular disease in Behçet's syndrome. In Yazici, H. & Yazici, Y. (Eds.), *Behçet's Syndrome* (pp. 115–133). New York, NY: Springer.

4. Seyahi, E., Fresko, I., & Yazici, H. (2010). Endothelial dysfunction and atherosclerosis in Behçet's syndrome. In Yazici, H. & Yazici, Y. (Eds.), *Behçet's Syndrome* (pp. 135–148). New York, NY: Springer.

5. Sarica-Kucukoglu, R., Akdag-Kose, A., KayabalI, M., Yazganoglu, K. D., Disci, R., Erzengin, D., & Azizlerli, G. (2006). Vascular involvement in Behçet's disease: a retrospective analysis of 2319 cases. *International journal of dermatology, 45(8)*, 919–921.

6. Fei, Y., Li, X., Lin, S., Song, X., Wu, Q., Zhu, Y... & Zhang, F. (2013). Major vascular involvement in Behçet's disease: a retrospective study of 796 patients. *Clinical rheumatology, 32(6)*, 845–852.

7. Saadoun, D., Asli, B., Wechsler, B., Houman, H., Geri, G., Desseaux, K... & Cacoub, P. (2012). Long-term outcome of arterial lesions in Behçet disease: a series of 101 patients. *Medicine, 91(1)*, 18–24.

8. Ugurlu, S., Seyahi, E., Oktay, V., Yigit, Z., Kucukoglu, S., & Yazici, H. (2013). Venous Claudication is a severe and frequent symptom in Behcet's syndrome. *Arthritis & Rheumatism, 65*(10 Supplement), S1117.

Behçet's and the lungs

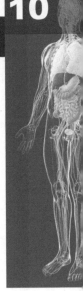

CHAPTER
10

55. What kinds of symptoms could point to Behçet's-related lung problems?

One out of every five Behçet's patients may have some type of lung (*pulmonary*) problem.[1] Some of these problems are more serious than others. Typical symptoms of lung involvement include a cough that won't go away, fever, shortness of breath (*dyspnea*), possible night sweats, and/or chest pain when you cough or take a breath. It's also possible, of course, that an illness other than Behçet's may be causing these symptoms, so it's important to check with your doctor.

If Behçet's affects a patient's pulmonary arteries, the results can be serious. Thankfully, this problem is rare. In a 20-year study of 387 Behçet's patients, only 10 men (and no women) developed pulmonary artery aneurysms (PAA).[4] A PAA is a balloon-like bulge in the wall of the pulmonary artery. Many BD patients with pulmonary artery problems have *hemoptysis*: they cough up blood or blood-tinged sputum,[2] although most bouts of hemoptysis are mild. "Massive" hemoptysis happens a lot less often, but it can be fatal in about half of the people who have it. A person with massive hemoptysis may cough up 500cc (two cups) or more of blood over a 24-hour period. PAAs eventually disappear in seven out of ten patients who develop them. They heal without complications in about 40% of the cases, and leave behind blockages or narrowed arteries in the other 60%.[2]

For clinicians: Since hemoptysis and other lung problems may get worse if an invasive test like a pulmonary angiogram is used to diagnose a PAA in Behçet's patients, researchers now suggest using a CT scan instead of an angiogram.[3]

If and when a patient's pulmonary-artery problem has gotten better and test results look normal again, about 40% of these patients may still cough up blood at times, have shortness of breath – especially with exercise—and/or chest pain. About 20% of patients relapse. Another 35% of the patients no longer have symptoms.[2]

56. What specific lung issues have been seen in Behçet's patients?[1,2,3,4]

The following are examples of lung problems seen in research studies with Behçet's patients (none of these problems is specific to Behçet's, and they can also occur in people with other illnesses): **recurring pneumonia**; **pneumonitis** (inflammation of lung tissue); **atelectasis** (one or more areas of the lung collapse or don't inflate properly); **bronchiectasis** (damage to the tubes carrying air in and out of the lungs; the tubes get flabby and scarred and lose their ability to clear out mucus); **bronchitis** (inflammation of the lining of the bronchial tubes); **cavitary lesions** (gas-filled cavities in lung tissue, usually in the lower lobes, within nodules or consolidations); **consolidations** (areas of lung tissue that have filled with fluid, with swelling or hardening of tissue); **emphysema** (damage to the air sacs in the lungs causing shortness of breath and difficulty in exhaling); **ground-glass opacities** (areas on a CT scan that look like glass that's been ground under a person's foot); **mediastinal lymphadenopathy** (swollen or enlarged lymph nodes in the *mediastinal compartment*—an area that includes the heart, esophagus, trachea, various nerves, and lymph nodes); **nodules** ("spots" on the lung that are about 1.5 inches in diameter or less and may be found in both lungs, most often in the inferior—lower—lobes); **pleural effusion** (the buildup of fluid in the thin space between the outside of the lungs and the chest wall); **pleural thickening** (scarring and/or thickening of the membrane that surrounds the lungs); **pleurisy or pleuritis** (inflammation of the *pleura*—the membrane that surrounds the lungs and also lines the inside of the chest wall); **pneumothorax** (collapsed lung, caused by the leakage of air into the space between the lungs and chest wall); **pulmonary arterial hypertension** (high blood pressure in the arteries of the lungs); **pulmonary fibrosis** (thickened and scarred tissue throughout the lungs); and **pulmonary hemorrhage** (sudden bleeding from the upper respiratory tract and/or the trachea).

As we saw in Question 55, problems with arteries in the lungs can be very serious for people with Behçet's. **Pulmonary artery aneurysms (PAA)** and **pulmonary artery thromboses (PAT,** clots) are the most lethal BD-related complications. They can appear in one or both lungs at the same time. A single patient may have several aneurysms or other blood vessel lesions at once.

Many BD patients with PAA also have deep-vein thrombosis (DVT) in a leg vein. It's rare, though, for these blood clots in the leg to travel to the lungs and cause an embolism, which is a sudden, dangerous blockage in a lung's artery. DVTs caused by Behçet's are "sticky" and usually stay put. As a result, it's important to find out if a BD patient has a pulmonary artery aneurysm before using anticoagulants to treat any blood clot in the leg or lungs.[1] Anticoagulation might cause a pulmonary artery aneurysm to get worse, with more coughing up of blood (hemoptysis), other complications, and—possibly—death.

In a 2012 research study, about a quarter of the original 47 BD patients with PAA and/or PAT eventually died from these complications. Immunosuppressants given with corticosteroids, though, can help to lower the death rates. Other treatment options include cyclophosphamide, azathioprine, infliximab, interferon, and mycophenolate mofetil.[2]

57. Can you have Behçet's-related lung problems even if you have normal test results?

Yes. For example, chest X-rays may be normal in some BD patients who have symptoms, including hemoptysis (coughing up blood). As a result, experts think it's important to do a CT scan of the lungs for any people with Behçet's who have breathing issues or unexplained fever.[2] Some research has linked unexplained fever to problems with a person's blood vessels.

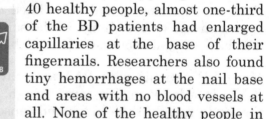

For patients who have limited-to-no symptoms and normal lung function tests, *expiratory high-resolution CT scans* (HRCT) may show *air trapping*, which suggests small airway disease. Air trapping is when a person tries to exhale but isn't able to get all air out of the lungs before taking another breath. Air is abnormally held back.

A *nail-fold capillaroscopy test* can help show if a Behçet's patient is dealing with microvascular damage to very small blood vessels in the body. In a 2014 study of 40 Behçet's patients and 40 healthy people, almost one-third of the BD patients had enlarged capillaries at the base of their fingernails. Researchers also found tiny hemorrhages at the nail base and areas with no blood vessels at all. None of the healthy people in the study had any of these issues.[5]

58. Can people with Behçet's develop BOOP? [6,7,8,9]

Yes. BOOP stands for *bronchiolitis obliterans organizing pneumonia*, also called *cryptogenic organizing pneumonia* (COP). BOOP can show up in diseases like lupus, rheumatoid arthritis and ankylosing spondylitis, as well as Behçet's. Many experts think BOOP is the lung's autoimmune response to injured tissue. BOOP may start with flu-like symptoms, fever, a dry cough, chest pain, and a shortness of breath when the person is active. In the beginning, it's sometimes mistaken for a lung infection; in those cases, treatment with antibiotics won't work. As BOOP gets worse, CT scans may show nodules, consolidations, and ground-glass opacities in the lung(s) (see Question 56 for definitions). A biopsy is the best way to confirm the diagnosis. Treatment is usually started with high-dose corticosteroids, often by IV. A slow oral taper over six months or more will help avoid relapses.

A personal Behçet's contact developed BOOP after breast-cancer radiation treatments and breast-sparing surgery. BOOP is different from radiation pneumonitis, the type of pneumonia that's caused by radiation treatments to the chest; in BOOP, opacities and consolidations may eventually be seen outside the radiated port area, and these problems may move around (migrate) to different locations. Administration of corticosteroids with a slow taper was critical for this patient's recovery.

References

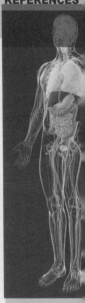

CHAPTER 10

1. Zhang, X., Dai, H., Ma, Z., Yang, Y., & Liu, Y. (2014). Pulmonary involvement in patients with Behçet's disease: Report of fifteen cases. *The clinical respiratory journal. Online first, doi:doi/10.1111/crj.12153.*

2. Seyahi, E., Melikoglu, M., Akman, C., Hamuryudan, V., Ozer, H., Hatemi, G... & Yazici, H. (2012). Pulmonary artery involvement and associated lung disease in Behçet disease: a series of 47 patients. *Medicine, 91(1)*, 35–48.

3. Erkan, F., Kiyan, E., & Tunaci, A. (2002). Pulmonary complications of Behçet's disease. *Clinics in chest medicine, 23(2)*, 493–503.

4. Kural-Seyahi, E., Fresko, I., Seyahi, N., Ozyazgan, Y., Mat, C., Hamuryudan, V., Yurdakul, S., & Yazici, H. (2003). The long-term mortality and morbidity of Behçet's syndrome: a 2-decade outcome survey of 387 patients followed at a dedicated center. *Medicine, 82(1)*, 60–76.

5. Aytekin, S., Yuksel, E. P., Aydin, F., Senturk, N., Ozden, M. G., Canturk, T., & Turanli, A. Y. (2014). Nailfold capillaroscopy in Behçet disease, performed using videodermoscopy. *Clinical and experimental dermatology, 39(4)*, 443–447.

6. Epler, G. R. (2001). Bronchiolitis obliterans organizing pneumonia. *Archives of internal medicine, 161(2)*, 158–164.

7. Erdogan, E., Demirkazik, F. B., Emri, S., & Firat, P. (2006). Organizing pneumonia after radiation therapy for breast cancer. *Diagnostic and interventional radiology (Ankara, Turkey), 12(3)*, 121–124.

8. Nanke, Y., Kobashigawa, T., Yamada, T., Kamatani, N., & Kotake, S. (2007). Cryptogenic organizing pneumonia in two patients with Behçet's disease. *Clinical and experimental rheumatology, 25(4) Suppl 45*, S103–6.

9. Rutherford, R. M., O'Keeffe, D., & Gilmartin, J. J. (2004). An unusual case of non-specific interstitial pneumonitis. *Respiration; international review of thoracic diseases, 71(2)*, 202–205.

Behçet's in families and children

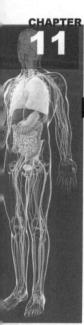

59. Is Behçet's genetic?

As we've seen in Question 1, Behçet's isn't inherited in the same way as diseases like hemophilia or sickle cell anemia. Genes may make it more likely a person would develop Behçet's, but these genes need a "trigger" to get the disease started. This trigger could be a bacterial infection, a virus, or something else in the environment. Researchers are still looking for the cause.

Even though genetics is just one piece of the Behçet's puzzle, a few features show that it plays an important part:[7]

- Behçet's appears to run in some (but not all) families.
- HLA-B51 is linked to some (but not all) cases.
- The disease is most common in a geographic area: along the old Silk Road trade routes.
- There is evidence of *genetic anticipation* in some children who have BD (see Question 62).
- Two large studies in 2010 found a strong link to the IL-10 and IL-23R genes in some BD patients. Changes in these genes may cause problems in a person's immune system.
- There's a significant *recurrence rate* for BD in some brothers and sisters and for identical twins in the same family. A recurrence rate is the chance that a disease will show up again in one or more blood relatives in a family.

Learn more about IL-10 and IL-23R here:
IL-10: http://ghr.nlm.nih.gov/gene/IL10
IL-23R: http://ghr.nlm.nih.gov/gene/IL23R
Read one of the genome-wide studies on IL-10 and IL-23R in Behçet's disease:
http://www.ncbi.nlm.nih.gov/pmc/articles/PMC2923807/pdf/nihms-214962.pdf

ON THE WEB

60. Can Behçet's be passed on to your children?

People who have Behçet's disease are often worried about passing it on to their children. Behçet's sometimes runs in families, but it's more common in certain ethnic groups than in others. For example, Turkish, Korean, and Jewish families seem to have higher numbers of affected blood relatives (18%, 15%, and 13%, respectively), while the lowest numbers are within Japanese and European families (2% and 1%).[1] In general around the world, though, three or four BD patients out of 100 will have other blood relatives with Behçet's.

If you've been diagnosed with Behçet's and you have a child who gets occasional oral ulcers, don't panic. One out of every four healthy people has recurrent mouth sores for no known reason. Other oral ulcers may be caused by infections, food allergies/ sensitivities, or nutritional deficiencies, like a low level of vitamin B12. The parent, child or brother/sister of a BD patient may also get a rare genital ulcer or a positive pathergy test result, but no other Behçet's symptoms.[3]

It's common for one or more types of autoimmune diseases— such as MS, lupus, or ulcerative colitis—to pop up in the families of autoimmune patients, including Behçet's patients. Some BD patients may even have an overlapping diagnosis of Behçet's and lupus or another disease.

61. Can more than one person in a family have Behçet's?

Yes. There have been published reports of people who have several blood relatives with Behçet's. When 137 Behçet's patients were asked about their relationship to other family members who had BD, 45 of the patients had brothers with Behçet's; 27 had sisters with BD; 14 had cousins with BD; 22 had mothers with BD; 11 had fathers with BD; 5 had parents with BD; 6 had daughters with BD; 9 had sons with BD; 13 had uncles or aunts with BD; and 2 had nephews or nieces with BD.[2]

There are reports of identical Turkish twins who are both HLA-B51 positive and diagnosed with Behçet's. Showing that there's more to a BD diagnosis than genetics, though, there's also a report of "discordant" identical twins: one twin who developed Behçet's while the other didn't. Both of these twins were HLA-B51 negative.[1] HLA-A2 and HLA-Cw16 are some other possible HLA results in families with BD but—just like HLA-B51—they're not required for a Behçet's diagnosis.

Some Behçet's symptom clusters may appear more often in families that have BD. For example, a 2012 report says that papulopustular skin lesions and arthritis tend to show up together more frequently in blood relatives with BD.[5]

Finally, when a person **under the age of 16** has been diagnosed with a complete case of Behçet's according to the ISG Classification Criteria (see Question 15), there's a higher chance of finding other people in the same family who also have BD. People diagnosed with BD as an *adult*, though, seem to have fewer affected relatives.[4]

62. What is "genetic anticipation," and how does it apply to Behçet's?

Genetic anticipation is when the symptoms of a genetic disease show up at a younger age in the child(ren) of a patient than they did in the patient himself, **and/or** when the disease has symptoms that are worse in that next generation.

Children with Behçet's who have other blood relatives with BD usually meet all of the ISG Classification Criteria for diagnosis (see Question 15) a full 10 years earlier than people who don't have Behçet's in the family.[4]

63. Do children with Behçet's have different symptoms than adults with Behçet's?

Most experts say Behçet's in children is similar to the disease in adults, but there are still some differences:

- Children with Behçet's have more abdominal pain than adults. They may also have diarrhea, constipation, small ulcers in the stomach, and/or intestinal inflammation and ulcers.
- Perianal (around the anus) ulcers are more common in children than adults.
- Children with Behçet's may have uveitis less often than adults, but it can be more severe. As a result, ophthalmologists who specialize in uveitis often use an aggressive approach to the treatment of Behçet's-related eye problems in children. The goal is to reduce inflammation as quickly as possible and avoid any vision loss.
- Young males may have a more severe case of Behçet's than young females, or than adults of either sex.
- While it doesn't happen often, children with **neuro-**Behçet's have a higher chance of developing a blood clot in the brain (cerebral venous sinus thrombosis or CVST)

than adults with neuro-BD. This problem may also raise the pressure of cerebrospinal fluid inside the skull. It can cause a very severe headache that happens suddenly or gets steadily worse over time. This headache may be the only symptom, or there could also be abnormal vision or stroke-like symptoms. When Behçet's affects the nervous system of adults, though, they usually have problems with inflammation instead of a blood clot: the brain and/ or spinal cord can get inflamed, and there may be a fever, headache and a very stiff neck. If the brainstem is affected, the person may have dizziness, hearing loss, double vision, difficulty speaking or moving, and/or drooping facial muscles. Since CVST is usually rare in children, **any** child with CVST should be checked for other Behçet's-type symptoms.

 If your child has uveitis, look at the Ocular Immunology and Uveitis Foundation's booklet, *Uveitis: A guide for teachers and parents*, at http://www.uveitis.org/patients/education/patient-guides. You can also order a free printed copy at the uveitis.org website.

64. What other Behçet's-related issues in children are especially important? [7,8,9,10]

- If children get Behçet's-related genital ulcers at all, they usually show up for the first time around puberty. The most common age range, though, is from 5 to 12.
- Children with genital ulcers, especially teenagers, are often told they have a sexually transmitted disease even though test results are negative. In addition, these children may be accused of hiding sexual activity from their parents. It's important to take a **full** medical history of any child with genital ulcers, keeping Behçet's in mind once other medical reasons for these ulcers have been ruled out.
- Behçet's can cause urinary tract infections as well as orchitis (inflammation of one or both testicles) and epididymitis (inflammation of a tube in the back of the testicle).
- Results of ESR (erythrocyte sedimentation rate or "sed rate") and CRP (C-reactive protein) tests can show if people have inflammation somewhere in their body. Some children and adults with Behçet's, however, may

have normal ESR and CRP levels even when they're having a flare-up of symptoms.

- It's possible for ulcers to be deep in the throat, causing pain, swelling, and trouble with swallowing. Some throat inflammations/ulcers are incorrectly labeled as tonsillitis.
- Headaches are as common in children with Behçet's as they are in adults with BD—up to 70% of BD patients have headaches on a regular basis. However, only a small number of headaches is actually caused by Behçet's-related neurological problems.
- Up to 50% of children with Behçet's have fevers on a regular basis.
- Joint pain is common in children with Behçet's and it often affects the knees, ankles, wrists, elbows, and shoulders. This pain may come and go and/or move from joint to joint. It can happen on both sides of the body or only on one side.

65. Will my child outgrow Behçet's at puberty?

Unfortunately, there's no medical proof that a child with Behçet's will outgrow it at puberty.

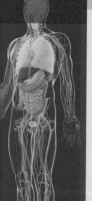

REFERENCES

References

CHAPTER 11

1. Fietta, P. (2005). Behçet's disease: familial clustering and immunogenetics. *Clinical and experimental rheumatology, 23(4 Suppl 38)*, S96-105. Available online at http://www.clinexprheumatol.org/article.asp?a=2733

2. Zeis, J. (2003). Behçet's disease in families. In *Essential Guide to Behçet's Disease* (pp. 95-100). Uxbridge, MA: Central Vision Press.

3. Gul, A., Inanc, M., Ocal, L., Aral, O., & Konice, M. (2000). Familial aggregation of Behçet's disease in Turkey. *Annals of the rheumatic diseases, 59(8)*, 622–625. Available online at http://ard.bmj.com/content/59/8/622.long

4. Kone-Paut, I., Geisler, I., Wechsler, B., Ozen, S., Ozdogan, H., Rozenbaum, M., & Touitou, I. (1999). Familial aggregation in Behçet's disease: high

frequency in siblings and parents of pediatric probands. *The Journal of pediatrics, 135(1),* 89–93.

5. Karaca, M., Hatemi, G., Sut, N., & Yazici, H. (2012). The papulopustular lesion/ arthritis cluster of Behçet's syndrome also clusters in families. *Rheumatology (Oxford, England), 51(6),* 1053–1060. Available online at http://rheumatology.oxfordjournals.org/content/51/6/1053.long

6. Kone-Paut, I., Darce-Bello, M., Shahram, F., Gattorno, M., Cimaz, R., Ozen, S., Cantarini, L., & PED-BD Intl Expert Committee. (2011). Registries in rheumatological and musculoskeletal conditions. Paediatric Behçet's disease: an international cohort study of 110 patients. One-year follow-up data. *Rheumatology (Oxford, England), 50(1),* 184–188. Available online at http://rheumatology.oxfordjournals.org/content/50/1/184.long

7. Ozen, S., & Eroglu, F. K. (2013). Pediatric-onset Behçet disease. *Current opinion in rheumatology, 25(5),* 636–642.

8. Kone-Paut, I., Yurdakul, S., Bahabri, S. A., Shafae, N., Ozen, S., Ozdogan, H., & Bernard, J. L. (1998). Clinical features of Behçet's disease in children: an international collaborative study of 86 cases. *The journal of pediatrics, 132(4),* 721–725.

9. Metreau-Vastel, J., Mikaeloff, Y., Tardieu, M., Kone-Paut, I., & Tran, T. A. (2010). Neurological involvement in paediatric Behçet's disease. *Neuropediatrics, 41(5),* 228–234.

10. Borlu, M., Uksal, U., Ferahbas, A., & Evereklioglu, C. (2006). Clinical features of Behçet's disease in children. *International journal of dermatology, 45(6),* 713–716.

Behçet's in pregnancy and postpartum

66. Do Behçet's symptoms get better or worse during pregnancy?

In general, Behçet's-related symptoms improve during pregnancy. In fact, symptoms get better—or totally stop—for around 7 out of every 10 pregnant women with BD.[1] The rest of the women either have flare-ups during pregnancy, or the symptoms they've had at the time of conception get worse. Some women also have one or more Behçet's-related symptoms during pregnancy that they've never had to deal with before.

According to a 2013 review,[1] oral ulcers are the most common symptom flare-up during pregnancy (57% of patients have

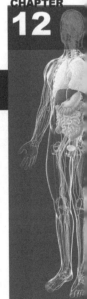

them). Genital ulcers are next (44%), followed by skin lesions (25%) and eye inflammation (6%), which is mostly uveitis. Any other typical BD symptoms, like joint pain, GI problems or neurological issues, can also happen in pregnancy.

A small number of women with Behçet's have vascular problems when pregnant, such as deep vein thrombosis (a blood clot in a vein deep in the body) or Budd–Chiari syndrome (a blockage of the hepatic veins that drain the liver). Some pregnant Behçet's patients have also developed rare cases of superior vena cava thrombosis, intracardiac thrombosis (both are heart-related blood clots) or dural sinus thrombosis (a blood clot in a vein that drains blood from the brain).

Each pregnancy can be different for a woman with Behçet's. While all symptoms may go away during one pregnancy, another pregnancy may have symptom flare-ups or complications. As a result, many specialists treat BD-related pregnancies as possible high-risk cases and watch them carefully.

67. Is there any information on pregnant women with Behçet's in the United States?

Yes, although it's based on an unpublished survey done by the author and given in a poster presentation at the 2006 International Conference on Behçet's Disease in Portugal.[3] In this survey, 65 American women with Behçet's shared what happened to them during their 204 pregnancies.

Symptoms got worse in one out of every four (22%) pregnant women with Behçet's who participated in the survey. Symptoms got better or disappeared completely in one-third of the US pregnancies (31%), while almost half of the women (46%) had symptoms that stayed at the same level during the pregnancy as they'd been when the women first got pregnant. This group also included women who'd had no symptoms when they got pregnant and stayed symptom-free for nine months.

Symptoms during pregnancy can be seen in Figure 12.1 and Table 12.1.

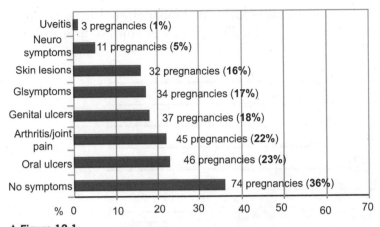

▲ Figure 12.1
Self-reported symptoms during pregnancies of 65 American women (204 pregnancies)
Source: J. Zeis, 2006

Table 12.1 Self-reported symptom details during pregnancies of 65 American women (204 pregnancies)

Symptom during pregnancy	Details
Neurological	Unclassified headaches (4 pregnancies); migraines (4); memory loss (3); coordination/balance problems (1); dizziness (1); double vision (1); loss of sensation from waist down (1); optic neuritis (1); tremors (1); weakness/numbness in legs (1).
Skin lesions	Raised red bumps on skin (6 pregnancies); folliculitis (3); clear, itchy, fluid-filled blisters on hands (2); cystic acne (2); unexplained rashes (2); large single bumps on legs (1); lesions on leg/trunk/upper arms (1); lichen planus (1); pustules (1); sores on buttocks/legs (1).
GI problems	Irritable bowel syndrome (6 pregnancies); severe abdominal cramping (4); severe vomiting (4); gastroesophageal reflux (GERD) (3); anal fistula (1); duodenitis (1); hiatal hernia (1); pain/mucous with stools (1); severe sore throat diagnosed as strep with negative strep test (1); unexplained diarrhea (1); unexplained lower right quadrant pain (1).

Behçet's-related symptoms happened most often during the first trimester (see Figure 12.2). This result is similar to a non-US study in 1997.[2]

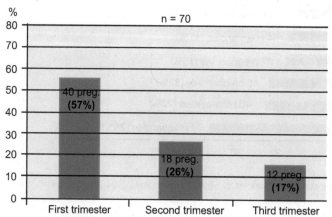

▲ **Figure 12.2**
Development of symptoms by trimester in American women with Behçet's (70 pregnancies)
Source: J. Zeis, 2006

Table 12.2 Self-reported symptoms that developed **after** deliveries of 65 American women in 204 pregnancies (including after miscarriage, stillbirth and voluntary termination)

Postpartum symptom	# of pregnancies	% of total pregnancies
Uveitis	7	3%
Neurological [a]	22	11%
No symptoms	27	13%
Skin lesions [b]	34	17%
GI symptoms [c]	36	18%
Genital ulcers	40	20%
Arthritis/joint pain	49	24%
Oral ulcers	54	27%

[a] Neuro = Severe headaches/migraines (4 pregnancies); peripheral neuropathy (3); seizures (2); stiff neck (3); coordination problems (2); short-term memory loss (2); balance problems (1); numbness in extremities (1); ocular migraines (1); optic neuritis (1); stroke (1); "swelling in brain" (1); TIAs (1).

[b] Skin lesions = Pustules (5); cystic acne (4); unexplained rashes (4); lichen planus (2); pityriasis rosea (2); red nodules on legs (2); erythema nodosum (1); painful red nodules on legs and groin (1); folliculitis (1); rash over entire body (1); painful genital sores/lumps, but no open ulcers (1).

[c] GI problems = Irritable bowel syndrome (6); gastric ulcerations (3); anal fistula (1); anal fissures (1); GERD (1); diarrhea (1); duodenitis (1); blood in stool (1); unexplained lower right quadrant pain (1).

There were several issues with this informal American survey: all symptoms were self-reported; there was no medical review of the women's records; there were no matched case-controls; there was no information on medications taken or other illnesses that the women had; and only 38% of women taking the survey used their medical records as a reference, while 58% relied on their memory. However, women who relied on their memory gave answers that were very close to the ones from women who used their medical records. This result suggests that women using memory alone were still able to give reliable responses.

ON THE WEB See the full results of the American survey on pregnancy and postpartum in women with BD: http://behcets.blogspot.com/2009/01/behcets-disease-and-pregnancypart-2.html

68. Does Behcet's cause problems with fertility?

Not according to a 2013 study on fertility in Behçet's patients.[4] The researchers defined infertility as not being able to conceive after one year of unprotected intercourse. They compared five large groups of people in their study: Behçet's patients who have major BD-related health problems; Behçet's patients with milder symptoms (for example, oral/genital ulcers); people with familial Mediterranean fever (FMF) or ankylosing spondylitis (two other diseases that can cause inflammation); and healthy people. There was no difference in the number of women with Behçet's who were able to get pregnant compared to women in the other groups. In addition, women with Behçet's were just as likely to get pregnant after being diagnosed as the women in the other groups. There was also no difference in the number of BD patients who were finally able to get pregnant, whether they used fertility treatments or not.

The researchers checked to see if common Behçet's medications, like azathioprine, cyclophosphamide, or colchicine have any effect on fertility. Of these three medications, only cyclophosphamide made it harder for Behçet's patients to get pregnant.[4] Other studies have found that sulfasalazine can affect male fertility,[5] and that NSAIDs (non-steroidal anti-inflammatory drugs like aspirin, ibuprofen, and naproxen) can affect ovulation in women. However, these problems go away when the medication is stopped.

69. Do women with Behçet's have more miscarriages than normal?

Women with Behçet's don't seem to have more miscarriages than healthy women. According to the American Pregnancy Association at americanpregnancy.org, up to one out of every four confirmed pregnancies in the United States (25%) ends in miscarriage. In a 2013 review article that looked at 279 pregnancies in non-US women with Behçet's, 25 (9%) of the pregnancies ended in miscarriage.[1] Miscarriage rates ranged from 0% to 21% of all pregnancies in these studies. A 2014 study in Turkey found no difference in miscarriage rates between women with and without BD.[4]

In an American survey of pregnant women with Behçet's, there were 20 miscarriages in 169 US pregnancies—a rate of 12%.[3] Seven additional US women with BD had a total of 35 miscarriages between them; their information wasn't included in the final tally because doctors never came up with a medical reason for the very high rate. With these totals included in the American survey, however, the miscarriage rate rose to 27%.

Regardless, all of the reported or published miscarriage rates for Behçet's pregnancies in the US and abroad fall within, or very close to, the normal 10-25% range.

70. What kinds of complications have been reported in Behçet's pregnancies?

In a 2013 study of pregnant women with Behçet's,[1] most of the women (84%) had no complications during pregnancy, while 12 women (16%) had issues that mostly included miscarriages and C-sections. The few serious complications included deep vein thrombosis (DVT: a blood clot in a vein deep in the body) with and without dural sinus thrombosis (a blood clot in the brain); two cases of pulmonary embolism (a blocked blood vessel in the lungs) and renal vein thrombosis (a blood clot in a vein that drains blood from the kidney); and thrombocytopenia (a low platelet count, which keeps the blood from clotting). The authors of the study warn that women with a history of vascular problems such as blood clots seem to have a higher chance of miscarriage.

Other complications in Behçet's pregnancies have been reported as individual cases.[3] They include pericarditis (inflammation of the sac surrounding the heart); thrombophlebitis (blood clot in one or more veins); preeclampsia (high blood pressure, usually after 20 weeks of pregnancy, with high protein levels in the urine, severe headaches and other serious issues); jaundice (yellowed skin, often from liver disease); Budd–Chiari syndrome (blocked veins draining blood from the liver); cerebral venous thrombosis (blood clot in the brain); superior vena cava thrombosis (blockage of the superior vena cava blood vessel in the chest, causing shortness of breath, with facial or arm swelling and other symptoms); intrauterine growth restriction (IUGR: when the baby doesn't grow at a normal rate during pregnancy and is smaller than expected); and fetal distress (low oxygen levels in the fetus).

Even though complications don't usually happen, most specialists would rather label a Behçet's pregnancy as high-risk so they're able to keep a close eye on any possible problems.

71. What Behçet's medications are safe to take during pregnancy and breastfeeding?

Please speak with your doctor and/or obstetrician **before you try to get pregnant**. Some medications are safe to take during pregnancy, some are questionable, and some should never be taken—even a few months before you try to conceive. Your medical history may also be different from other women with Behçet's, which may change the medicines you're able to take. Always speak with your doctor before adding to or changing any of your dosing schedules, even if you're trying "natural" products or supplements.

 ON THE WEB

Pregnancy and medicines fact sheet from WomensHealth.gov For more information on pregnancy and medications, see Chapter 12 reference numbers 5, 6, 8, 9, and 10.

72. What is neonatal Behçet's?[7]

Neonatal Behçet's is when BD-type symptoms appear in a newborn, either right after birth or often within 7-10 days. These symptoms may go away on their own after a few days, or they may last for weeks. Temporary neonatal Behçet's health problems can include mouth, throat, and/or genital ulcers; vomiting; diarrhea; skin lesions; fever; pathergy; leukocytosis (a high white blood cell count); intrauterine growth restriction

(IUGR: when the fetus doesn't grow at a normal rate and is smaller than expected); weight loss; and a failure to thrive.

After ruling out possible infections, doctors often use corticosteroids to clear up the baby's symptoms. In most cases, the mother of a child with neonatal Behçet's has already been diagnosed with Behçet's before conception and has dealt with BD symptoms during her pregnancy.

Why does neonatal Behçet's happen? Experts think the mother's antibodies may cross over to the placenta during pregnancy and it's the cause of temporary Behçet's symptoms in a newborn. Once the mother's antibodies disappear after a few weeks, the baby's Behçet's is also gone; it may never show up again.

REFERENCES 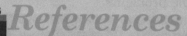 *References*

CHAPTER 12

1. Noel, N., Wechsler, B., Nizard, J., Costedoat-Chalumeau, N., Boutin, d. u. . L. T., Dommergues, M., Vauthier-Brouzes, D., Cacoub, P., & Saadoun, D. (2013). Behcet's disease and pregnancy. *Arthritis and rheumatism, 65(9)*, 2450–2456.

2. Bang, D., Chun, Y. S., Haam, I. B., Lee, E. S., & Lee, S. (1997). The influence of pregnancy on Behcet's disease. *Yonsei medical journal, 38(6)*, 437–443. Available online at http://www.eymj.org/Synapse/Data/PDFData/0069YMJ/ymj-38-437.pdf

3. Zeis, J. A. (2006). Behcet's disease, pregnancy and postpartum in the United States. *Clinical and Experimental Rheumatology, 24*(Supp. 42), S-41.

4. Saygin, C., Uzunaslan, D., Hatemi, G., Tascilar, K., & Yazici, H. (2013). Fertility in Behcet's syndrome: structured interview in a multidisciplinary center. *Arthritis & Rheumatism, 65*(10 Supplement), S1121.

5. Bernas, B. L. (2014). *Effects of anti-inflammatory and immunosuppressive drugs on gonadal function in men with rheumatic diseases*, at http://www.uptodate.com/contents/effects-of-antiinflammatory-andimmunosuppressive-drugs-on-gonadal-function-in-men-with-rheumaticdiseases

6. Arthritis Foundation (2011). *Arthritis medications in pregnancy: what's safe, what's not?* Available online at http://www.arthritistoday.org/about-arthritis/arthritis-and-your-health/pregnancy/safe-medications-during-pregnancy.php

7. Jog, S., Patole, S., Koh, G., & Whitehall, J. (2001). Unusual presentation of neonatal Behcets disease. *American journal of perinatology, 18(5)*, 287–292.

8. Raja, H., Matteson, E. L., Michet, C. J., Smith, J. R., & Pulido, J. S. (2012). Safety of Tumor Necrosis Factor Inhibitors during Pregnancy and Breastfeeding. *Translational vision science & technology, 1(2)*, 6. Available online at http://www.ncbi.nlm.nih.gov/pmc/articles/PMC3763882/pdf/i2164-2591-1-2-6.pdf

9. Marchioni, R. M., & Lichtenstein, G. R. (2013). Tumor necrosis factor alpha inhibitor therapy and fetal risk: a systematic literature review. *World journal of gastroenterology: WJG, 19(17)*, 2591–2602. Available online at http://www.ncbi.nlm.nih.gov/pmc/articles/PMC3645377/pdf/WJG-19-2591.pdf

10. Ostensen, M., Lockshin, M., Doria, A., Valesini, G., Meroni, P., Gordon, C., Brucato, A., & Tincani, A. (2008). Update on safety during pregnancy of biological agents and some immunosuppressive anti-rheumatic drugs. *Rheumatology (Oxford, England)*, iii28-31. Available online at http://rheumatology.oxfordjournals.org/content/47/suppl_3/iii28.full.pdf+html

Treatments for Behçet's disease

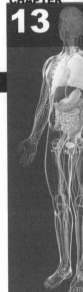

CHAPTER 13

73. Which medications work best for which symptoms?

Behçet's experts don't always agree on the best way to treat symptoms, but at least the old 1980s "wait and see" approach for handling some of them has changed. Eye involvement is a good example. Most uveitis specialists now agree it's key to get eye inflammation under control before it permanently damages a patient's vision, even if only one eye is inflamed. Thankfully, many of the eye-treatment medications that are taken by mouth or injected can also work on inflammation in other parts of the body. That's just one of many reasons for specialists to stay in touch and work together to control your symptoms.

Not only are doctors treating Behçet's symptoms earlier, they've also started using more aggressive treatment options in the last decade,[1] including drugs in combination.

Some guidelines have been put together by Behçet's experts around the world for the best ways to treat certain symptoms:

- **Overview of BD symptoms/ treatment:** The *EULAR recommendations for the management of Behçet's disease* (2008)[2] are available online at http://ard.bmj.com/ content/67/12/1656.full.pdf+html
- **GI symptoms:** *The 2nd edition of consensus statements for the diagnosis and management of intestinal Behçet's disease: indication of anti-TNF alpha monoclonal antibodies* (2014)[3] is available online at http://www.ncbi. nlm.nih.gov/pmc/articles/PMC3895195/ pdf/535_2013_Article_872.pdf
- **Neurological symptoms:** *Diagnosis and management of neuro-Behçet's disease: international consensus recommendations* (2013)[4] is available online at http://link. springer.com/content/pdf/10.1007%2Fs00415-013-7209-3. pdf

Table 13.1 shows systems of the body and/or symptoms, and the drugs that work best in each area. Table 13.2 lists drugs alphabetically along with their uses. Topical treatments have already been covered in Question 21. **Please note:** All drugs listed in this chapter may carry different names outside of the United States. Some of the drugs may be available only by prescription in some countries, while being available over the counter (or after speaking with the pharmacist) in others. Finally, people taking anti-TNF medications like Enbrel, Remicade and Humira risk the development of tuberculosis and dangerous systemic fungal infections. Ask your doctor for more information.

Table 13.1 Overview of Behçet's symptoms and most-used treatments. **May not include all possible options.**

Area of BD involvement	Medications used
Oral/genital ulcers and/or skin lesions	*For single, occasional lesions:* see Question 21. *For moderate to severe lesions:* alemtuzumab; antibiotics (tetracycline, minocycline, penicillin); anti-TNF (infliximab); apremilast (awaiting FDA approval for BD); azathioprine; colchicine; dapsone; interferon alpha; methylprednisolone injected into the lesion; pentoxifylline; rebamipide; sucralfate; thalidomide.
Eyes	*Anterior uveitis/iritis:* corticosteroid eye drops; dilation drops to keep pupil moving; oral prednisone. *Posterior uveitis/retinal vasculitis/severe eye disease:* adalimumab; alemtuzumab; azathioprine (often with systemic corticosteroids for posterior uveitis; also used to prevent development of new eye disease); cyclosporine A or infliximab with azathioprine and corticosteroids **OR** interferon alpha with or without steroids; methotrexate; mycophenolate mofetil (MMF); rituximab.
GI involvement	6-MP; azathioprine; corticosteroids; infliximab; mesalazine (for esophageal ulcers); methotrexate; rebamipide; sulfasalazine; tacrolimus; thalidomide; thiopurine.
Joint pain/arthritis	Colchicine; colchicine and azathioprine; interferon alpha; NSAIDS like piroxicam (Feldene); hydroxychloroquine (Plaquenil); anti-TNF meds (e.g. infliximab, etanercept, rituximab). Other possibilities include alemtuzumab (Campath); certolizumab (Cimzia), golimumab (Simponi) and leflunomide (Arava).

Area of BD involvement	Medications used
Neurological involvement	**Note:** Cyclosporine A is **not** recommended for BD patients who have neurological involvement, unless it's also needed for severe eye disease and if the benefits outweigh possible neurological risks. *For first-time parenchymal symptoms:* methylprednisolone IV pulse for 3-10 days, followed with tapered oral corticosteroid up to 6 months; methylprednisolone IV pulse and azathioprine; azathioprine alone; cyclophosphamide; interferon alpha; methotrexate, followed with folic acid to reduce nausea; anti-TNF meds. *For parenchymal relapse:* First-line treatment is azathioprine. Next try mycophenolate mofetil; then methotrexate and cyclophosphamide. *If treatment is ineffective or relapse is aggressive:* interferon alpha or anti-TNF meds. *For cerebral venous sinus thrombosis (CVST/CVT):* use corticosteroids; don't use anticoagulants until systemic aneurysms are ruled out.
Vascular	*Deep vein thrombosis (DVT):* azathioprine; corticosteroids; cyclophosphamide or cyclosporine A. *For PA or PAA:* cyclophosphamide and corticosteroids or infliximab; IV steroid pulse with oral steroids afterwards.

Table 13.2 Medications used to treat Behçet's symptoms, listed alphabetically. **This list does not include all possible options or warnings. Ask your doctor about all side effects, drug interactions, and use during pregnancy.**

Generic med (Brand name)	Used to treat
Acetaminophen (Tylenol)	Minor aches and pains and fever. Often combined with other drugs for extra pain relief. Also called paracetamol outside the U.S., Canada, and Japan.
Adalimumab (Humira)	Oral/genital lesions; eyes, GI lesions; joints/arthritis; neuro-BD; vascular problems; may be given with methotrexate. **Note:** Adalimumab increases the risk for serious infections, including tuberculosis (TB) and dangerous fungal infections; test for TB before starting.
Alemtuzumab (Campath 1-H)	Very limited trials have shown good results on uveitis. A trial in 18 BD patients with multiple symptoms showed remission of all symptoms in 13 patients (72%) within six months. At average 25-month follow-up, 10 were in stable remission; six of them needed no other meds for remission, four needed additional immunosuppression to maintain remission.[9]
Anakinra (Kineret)	May help give prompt relief for many BD-related symptoms, but in 2013 report (Cantarini, Vitale et al.), average time to relapse of one or more symptoms was 29 weeks. **Note:** Shouldn't be taken with TNF inhibitors (adalimumab, etanercept and infliximab).
Apremilast (Otezla)	Oral/genital lesions; awaiting FDA approval for BD.

(Contd.)

Generic med (Brand name)	Used to treat
Azathioprine (Imuran)	Retinal vasculitis/eye lesions; oral/genital lesions; venous thrombosis; arteritis; joint pain; GI symptoms (given with thalidomide or infliximab); chronic progressive CNS lesions (in combination with corticosteroids). Can help prevent development of new eye disease.
Canakinumab (Ilaris)	Hard-to-treat uveitis and retinal vasculitis; other system problems.
Certolizumab (Cimzia)	Joint pain/arthritis; GI symptoms. **Note:** Certolizumab increases the risk for all types of infections, including tuberculosis (TB); test for TB before starting.
Chlorambucil (Leukeran)	Retinal vasculitis; chronic progressive CNS lesions; venous thrombosis; arteritis.
Colchicine (Colcrys)	Oral/genital lesions; joint pain/arthritis; pseudofolliculitis; erythema nodosum. **Note:** May cause severe diarrhea in some patients when starting; start slowly and work up to standard dose.
Contraceptives	Sometimes effective for women who flare around menstruation. May help with oral/genital lesions; erythema nodosum.
Corticosteroids	Used for many Behçet's symptoms and often taken with immunosuppressive meds to lower the amount of steroid needed for treatment ("steroid-sparing"). **Note:** Due to serious long-term side effects, use corticosteroids only for severe BD symptoms or life-threatening complications where benefits outweigh long-term risks.

Generic med (Brand name)	Used to treat
Cyclophosphamide (Cytoxan)	Retinal vasculitis; vascular problems (venous thrombosis, PAA, superior vena cava thrombosis, systemic arterial involvement); parenchymal CNS lesions; Budd-Chiari syndrome. **Note:** May cause serious birth defects.
Cyclosporine A (Neoral)	Uveitis; vascular problems (venous thrombosis). **Note:** May trigger or worsen neuro-Behçet's symptoms. Do not use in patients with neuro-BD unless it's also needed to treat severe eye disease and the benefits outweigh possible neurological risks. Don't eat grapefruit or drink grapefruit juice because it raises the amount of cyclosporine absorbed by your body.
Dapsone	Oral/genital lesions; erythema nodosum; acneiform skin lesions; papulopustular skin lesions; pseudofolliculitis.
Etanercept (Enbrel)	Oral/genital lesions; eyes; arthritis/joint pain; nodular skin lesions; papulopustular skin lesions; superior vena cava syndrome; Budd-Chiari syndrome. May be given with methotrexate. **Note:** Etanercept increases the risk for serious infections, including tuberculosis (TB) and dangerous fungal infections; test for TB before starting.
Gevokizumab (XOMA)	Eyes (treatment-resistant uveitis and retinal vasculitis).
Golimumab (Simponi)	Joint pain/arthritis. **Note:** Golimumab increases the risk for serious infections, including tuberculosis (TB) and dangerous fungal infections; test for TB before starting.

(Contd.)

Generic med (Brand name)	Used to treat
Hydroxychloroquine (Plaquenil)	Joint pain/arthritis. **Note:** Visual (retinal) side effects are rare with this drug, but can be serious.
Infliximab (Remicade)	Oral/genital lesions; eyes (usually given with azathioprine and/or cyclosporine A; or may be directly injected); arthritis/joint pain; GI problems (abdominal pain, rectal bleeding, GI ulcers and fistulae); neuro-Behçet's (new onset, relapsing or chronic progressive); vascular problems (superior vena cava syndrome, PAA). May be given with methotrexate. **Note:** Infliximab increases the risk for serious infections, including tuberculosis (TB) and dangerous fungal infections; test for TB before starting.
Interferon alpha	Eyes; oral/genital lesions; treatment-resistant joint pain/ arthritis; papulopustular skin lesions; parenchymal neuro-BD symptoms. **Note**: Don't combine with azathioprine—may cause myelosuppression (lowered ability of bone marrow to make blood cells).
Leflunomide (Arava)	Joint pain/arthritis. **Note:** May cause serious birth defects; this effect may last up to two years after you stop taking it.
Mesalazine	Esophageal ulcers.
Methotrexate (Rheumatrex)	Retinal vasculitis; joint pain/arthritis; chronic progressive neuro-Behçet's lesions. Folic acid tablets taken after methotrexate can reduce nausea.
MMF (CellCept)	(Mycophenolate Mofetil). Oral/genital lesions and CNS involvement.

Generic med (Brand name)	Used to treat
NSAIDs	Such as: aspirin; celecoxib (Celebrex); ibuprofen (Motrin); naproxen (Aleve); indomethacin (Indocin); ketorolac (Toradol); and piroxicam (Feldene). For general pain relief; joint pain/arthritis; oral/genital lesions.
Pentoxifylline (Trental)	Oral/genital ulcers; joint pain; fatigue; pseudofolliculitis; erythema nodosum.
Rebamipide	Oral/genital lesions; GI lesions.
Rituximab (Rituxan)	Retinal vasculitis.
Sucralfate (Carafate)	Suspension. Use for oral and esophageal ulcers.
Sulfasalazine (Azulfidine)	GI symptoms; joint pain/arthritis.
Tacrolimus (FK-506, Prograf)	Eyes.
Thalidomide (Thalomid)	For severe oral/genital lesions; GI lesions; follicular and papulopustular skin lesions. **Note**: Causes birth defects and may cause irreversible peripheral neuropathy.
Tocilizumab (Actemra)	Joint pain/arthritis; eyes; parenchymal neuro-BD.
Topiramate (Topamax)	Helps prevent migraines if taken daily.

74. Why can't I use prednisone all the time if it works so well?

It's easy to have a love-hate relationship with oral prednisone and high-dose IV steroids. There's no question this type of medication works quickly on almost any symptom you can name. It doesn't take long, though, for the hate to start. There are many possible side effects, and if you're on prednisone for weeks

Read patients' reviews of different medications
ON THE WEB Sometimes you just need to hear if certain drugs have worked for other people and whether or not they've had side effects. *Ask a Patient* hardly ever has ratings from people with Behçet's, but the compiled information is still helpful. Go to http://www.askapatient.com.

or months, you'll probably deal with some of them. Prednisone can cause trouble sleeping, make you gain weight, create a puffy "moon" face with fat deposits that cause a hump on the back of the neck, cause problems with healing and infections, lead to bruising and thin skin, cause mood swings, lead to steroid-caused diabetes and problems with the adrenal glands (adrenal glands release hormones—like adrenaline—in response to stress), and cause thinning of the bones (osteoporosis), cataracts, and glaucoma.

Caution: Never stop prednisone suddenly if you've been taking it for more than a few days. Your body needs time to get used to lower doses, so your doctor has to slowly taper the amount. In the same way, don't decide on your own to start taking prednisone for symptoms if you have pills left over from an old prescription. Talk about it with your doctor first! Depending on your current symptoms or overall health, you may need to take a different medication instead.

75. Will immunosuppressive medications make my hair fall out or lead to cancer?

Hair loss: There's less chance of hair loss in the lower doses used for treating rheumatic diseases like Behçet's. Drugs that may cause thinning hair in some (but not all) patients include azathioprine (Imuran), celecoxib (Celebrex), colchicine (Colcrys), cyclophosphamide (Cytoxan), infliximab (Remicade), interferon alpha, mesalazine (Pentasa), methotrexate, leflunomide (Arava), high blood pressure medications like propranolol (Inderal), and blood thinners like heparin. Once these medications are stopped, hair usually grows back.

Cancer: It's hard for researchers to prove a definite link between taking immunosuppressive drugs and getting cancer years later. In some cases, they're not sure if cancer is being caused by the severe inflammation of the disease itself or by the drugs being used to treat it. Also, most research studies have looked at the link to cancer in other diseases (not Behçet's) and in people who've had an organ transplant that require high immunosuppressant doses. As a result, there's no guarantee that people with BD would have the same outcomes. Some general findings have come up, though, in studies of rheumatoid arthritis:[7]

- Cyclophosphamide (Cytoxan) has the greatest risk of causing lymphoma, leukemia, and bladder cancer over the long term. Experts recommend using it for no more than six months, and only in life-threatening or organ-threatening situations.
- Methotrexate *may* create a higher risk of lymphoma in some people with rheumatic diseases.
- Azathioprine users may have a higher risk of lymphoma and leukemia.
- Anti-TNF drugs like infliximab, etanercept, and adalimumab don't seem to raise the overall risk of developing cancer, except for non-melanoma skin cancer.
- Rituximab seems safe so far. It's being suggested as a possible treatment for rheumatoid arthritis patients who have a history of cancer, but not for people with a history of non-melanoma skin cancer.
- Up to 25% of cancers in people taking anti-TNF drugs like infliximab, etanercept, and adalimumab usually show up in the first 12 weeks of treatment. Full cancer and skin screening should take place before starting these drugs.

ON THE WEB Get more information on the risk of cancer when immunosuppressives are used to treat uveitis: *Long-term risk of malignancy among patients treated with immunosuppressive agents for ocular inflammation: A critical assessment of the evidence* (2008) is available at http://www.ncbi.nlm.nih.gov/pmc/articles/PMC2614443/pdf/nihms81532.pdf

76. Do Behçet's patients have more complications after surgery than normal?

In general, yes—but it may depend on how active your Behçet's symptoms are when it's time for surgery. A 2007 study found that BD patients who have a positive pathergy test result close to surgery have a higher chance of problems after the operation.[8] These problems can show up after one out of every three surgeries and for up to 16 months afterwards. Complications occur most often within six months of the operation. They also happen more often after vascular surgeries (like heart valve replacements and aneurysm grafts) than nonvascular operations (like appendectomies, hysterectomies and intestinal perforations). See Question 41 for information about problems with BD-related GI surgery.

Types of complications seen in the 2007 study include surgical wounds that break open, infections, and grafts that fail or become blocked. By giving immunosuppressive meds along with steroids after an operation, there's less chance of these problems developing over time. It may help to use immunosuppressives before surgery, too, to quiet any flare that's going on— although some vascular surgeries may still have to take place on an emergency basis when symptoms are active. Cataract surgery is usually safe in BD patients whose eyes have been quiet for at least three months.

77. How can I find out about clinical trials for Behçet's?

Clinical trials help researchers figure out new ways to prevent, diagnose or treat diseases. Researchers are always looking for volunteers to try new treatments before they're approved by the FDA and used by doctors or sold in drugstores. You can look online to find available clinical trials for Behçet's. These trials may be taking place anywhere in the world, not just in the United States.

First, go to www.clinicaltrials.gov. Under "Search for Studies," type "Behçet's" and choose the box for "Include only open studies." While there were thousands of clinical trials going on for breast cancer research at the time of this writing, only 15 clinical trials were actively looking for Behçet's patients. It shows how few people/groups are doing research into Behçet's. Bookmark the clinicaltrials.gov Website and go back to it every few weeks. You never know when a researcher might be working on the BD problem that affects you the most.

78. Is bone marrow (stem cell) transplant a possible treatment for Behçet's?

Yes, but the procedure is risky, very expensive (at least $400,000 USD if you use your own stem cells), time-consuming, and it probably won't be covered by your health insurance if you live in the United States. Some BD patients may feel it's worth the risk and cost, though, if they have severe or life-threatening symptoms that haven't been helped by other treatments.

References

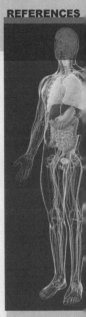

CHAPTER 13

1. Turkstra, F., van Vugt, R. M., Dijkmans, B. A., Yazici, Y., & Yazici, H. (2012). Results of a questionnaire on the treatment of patients with Behçet's syndrome: a trend for more intensive treatment. *Clinical and experimental rheumatology, 30(3 Suppl 72)*, S10–13.

2. Hatemi, G., Silman, A., Bang, D., Bodaghi, B., Chamberlain, A. M., Gul, A., Houman, M. H...& Yazici, H. (2008). EULAR recommendations for the management of Behçet disease. *Annals of the rheumatic diseases, 67(12)*, 1656–1662. Available online at http://ard.bmj.com/content/67/12/1656.full.pdf+html

3. Hisamatsu, T., Ueno, F., Matsumoto, T., Kobayashi, K., Koganei, K., Kunisaki, R., Hirai, F...& Hibi, T. (2014). The 2nd edition of consensus statements for the diagnosis and management of intestinal Behçet's disease: indication of anti-TNF alpha monoclonal antibodies. *Journal of gastroenterology, 49(1)*, 156–162. Available online at http://www.ncbi.nlm.nih.gov/pmc/articles/PMC3895195/pdf/535_2013_Article_872.pdf

4. Kalra, S., Silman, A., Akman-Demir, G., Bohlega, S., Borhani-Haghighi, A., Constantinescu, C. S., Siva, A...& Al-Araji, A. (2013). Diagnosis and management of Neuro-Behçet's disease: international consensus recommendations. *Journal of neurology, published online first at* http://www.ncbi.nlm.nih.gov/pmc/articles/PMC4155170/

5. Cantarini, L., Vitale, A., Scalini, P., Dinarello, C. A., Rigante, D., Franceschini, R...& Cimaz, R. (2013). Anakinra treatment in drug-resistant Behçet's disease: a case series. *Clinical rheumatology, Epub ahead of print, 2013 Dec 5.*

6. Sanchez-Cano, D., Callejas-Rubio, J. L., Ruiz-Villaverde, R., Rios-Fernandez, R., & Ortego-Centeno, N. (2013). Off-label uses of anti-TNF therapy in three frequent disorders: Behçet's disease, sarcoidosis, and noninfectious uveitis. *Mediators of inflammation, 286857*. Available online at http://www.ncbi.nlm.nih.gov/pmc/articles/PMC3747407/pdf/MI2013-286857.pdf

7. Turesson, C., & Matteson, E. L. (2013). Malignancy as a comorbidity in rheumatic diseases. *Rheumatology (Oxford, England), 127(1)*, 5–14.

8. Park, M. C., Hong, B. K., Kwon, H. M., & Hong, Y. S. (2007). Surgical outcomes and risk factors for postoperative complications in patients with Behcet's disease. *Clinical rheumatology, 26(9)*, 1475–1480.

9. Lockwood, C. M., Hale, G., Waldman, H., & Jayne, D. R. (2003). Remission induction in Behçet's disease following lymphocyte depletion by the anti-CD52 antibody CAMPATH 1-H. *Rheumatology (Oxford, England), 42(12)*, 1539–1544. Available online at http://rheumatology. oxfordjournals.org/content/42/12/1539.full.pdf+html

CHAPTER
14 *Disability benefits and prognosis*

79. Is it hard to get Social Security disability benefits for Behçet's in the United States?

Yes, but it's not impossible. The whole process, from the time you apply until the time you're approved (or denied at your last appeal), can take anywhere from a few months to a couple of years or more.

In 2002, the Social Security Administration (SSA) finally added Behçet's disease to its official List of Impairments, under the "Immune Systems/Inflammatory Arthritis" category. Being added to the list, though, doesn't mean automatic approval for disability payments. Only one out of every three disability applications (~38%) is approved the first time it's submitted, whether the person has Behçet's or any other illness.[1] The rest of the applications are turned down for a host of reasons, like the impairment isn't expected to last for 12 months or more; the impairment isn't severe; the applicant is able to do the usual past work; the applicant is able to do another type of work; or the applicant hasn't worked enough hours recently to qualify for benefits.

What's the difference between SSI (Supplemental Security Income) and SSDI (Social Security Disability Income)? Learn more here: http://www.ssa.gov/disability/

ON THE WEB

Any applicants that are turned down have the right to appeal, and this next step is called "reconsideration." It gives you a chance to offer more evidence and try to prove your case, but almost none of the applicants who appeal at this stage get approved for benefits—only about eight out of every 100 who apply.[1]

People who've been turned down at the reconsideration phase need to go before an Administrative Law Judge at one of the SSA's Offices of Disability Adjudication and Review (ODAR) for their next appeal. It may take 12–18 more months before this hearing is scheduled and the judge makes a decision. By this time, many applicants have hired a disability lawyer or advocate to help them. The good news is that about three out of every four people who see a judge (72%) are finally approved for payments.[1]

If you've hired a disability lawyer or advocate, you won't have to pay him or her unless you're finally approved for benefits. Payments would come out of any back-pay settlement, which dates back to the time you first applied. As of 2014, the standard lawyer/advocate fee is 25% of your back-pay settlement, up to a maximum of $6000.

Behçet's patients who were approved for disability benefits in the United States offer this advice:

- Behçet's symptoms come and go on a regular basis. Include on your symptom list **all** health issues that you face, even if they don't affect you every day.
- Don't sugarcoat your medical condition or downplay its effect on your life or your daily activities. The SSA can't make a decision on your case unless they have as much information as possible.

Appeals and reconsideration
The SSA is trying out a new system (the "Prototype" test) in 10 states. They've gotten rid of the reconsideration phase of appeals in these states on a trial basis to see if it improves the process. People who've been turned down for benefits on their first try can go straight to the next stage—a hearing before an Administrative Law Judge at one of the SSA's Offices of Disability Adjudication and Review (ODAR). The states in the Prototype trial are Alabama, Alaska, California (LA North and LA West branches), Colorado, Louisiana, Michigan, Missouri, New Hampshire, New York, and Pennsylvania. As of 2014, there's no word on how long this trial will continue. Get more information here: https://secure.ssa.gov/poms.nsf/lnx/0412015100

Finding a US disability lawyer or advocate
The best option is to join one or more online Behçet's support groups and ask if anyone can recommend a disability lawyer or advocate who helped them get approval for benefits. Another option is to contact the National Organization of Social Security Claimants' Representatives at http://www.nosscr.org or the Alliance of Professional Health Advocates (APHA) at http://www.advoconnection.com

- Don't be embarrassed to include any psychological problems you might have. They can be just as disabling as physical problems.
- If your claim is denied, you have the right to look at your Social Security file, including doctors' reports and other summaries of your case. Look for any mistakes because they may help with your appeal.

If you want to apply online for US disability benefits, go to https://secure.ssa.gov/iClaim/dib.

80. Is it true that Behçet's "burns out" in some patients as they get older?

Yes, it may happen for some—but not all—Behçet's patients. One of the longest studies on Behçet's disease looked at the health of a group of BD patients after 20 years.[1] The researchers got these results:

- Behçet's symptoms are at their worst for many patients during the first few years (usually in the patient's 20s or 30s).
- The worst eye damage and vision loss usually happens during the first seven years of BD symptoms. There's a better outcome if treatment is started at the first sign of eye involvement. Behçet's patients who have eye problems at a later stage of their disease still need treatment, but overall, they tend to keep more vision and have a better visual outcome.
- After 20 years, three out of five patients have so few symptoms that they wouldn't be given a Behçet's diagnosis. This is especially true for people whose BD started with skin lesions, oral or genital ulcers, and joint pain/arthritis.
- Even though Behçet's may burn out in many patients, that's not the case for everybody. People with central nervous system involvement and/or major blood vessel disease, like aneurysms, blood clots, and blockages, may have a tougher time over the long haul. That's especially true for young males.

The long-term study that came up with these results took place in Turkey. However, a newer 2014 study from one of the original authors says you shouldn't assume these results would apply to other parts of the world, like the United States and Western Europe. In fact, there are some big differences between BD patients in Turkey and the United States:[3]

- Many more women were in the US study than the one in Turkey. Ninety-nine out of 112 participants in the United States were women [88%], while only 65 out of 107 participants in Turkey were women [61%].
- Patients in the United States have less blindness and vascular involvement than patients in Turkey.
- Neurologic problems are much more common in the United States than in Turkey; they happen in about one out of every five US patients. In Turkey, only three out of every 100 BD patients has neurologic symptoms. In this study, "neurologic problems" are defined as either dural sinus thrombosis or white matter lesions on an MRI scan.
- Ulcers in the intestines happen in about four out of every 10 US patients, which is higher than reported in other studies. In this particular study, *no* Turkish patients had GI ulcers.
- Women with Behçet's in the United States report a worse quality of life and more active disease symptoms than patients in Turkey.
- Since many more US women than men have Behçet's in this study, it suggests that US-based *female* BD patients may be bearing the burden of serious neurological and GI problems. This sharply contrasts with the profile of *young men* in Silk Road countries having the most serious problems.

The study's authors raise these questions: Is the underlying cause of Behçet's different in each of these countries? Are we talking about the same disease in each country, or something different?

81. A lot of Behçet's patients who post on social networks seem really ill. Am I going to be that sick someday, too?

Probably not. In one of the only published surveys of BD patients' experiences in the United States, 245 members of the American Behçet's Disease Association rated how bad they felt their symptoms were. Almost seven out of every ten patients (69%) said they had "mild" or "moderate" symptoms.[4] The rest said their symptoms were severe. People with the most severe symptoms usually had the longest lag time between the start of their symptoms and diagnosis/treatment—up to 12 years in some cases. Three out of every four patients said they didn't need other people to help them on a regular basis; many felt it only took a "minimal" amount of effort to care for themselves every day.

Posts in online Behçet's support groups may make it seem like all of the group members (therefore all BD patients) are very ill, but you have to remember that very few members of online groups actually participate. Most people in these groups stay in the background to learn as much as possible, but they may be shy about posting. The people who post most often usually have serious symptoms that they want to compare with other patients, or they need emotional support for difficult times with friends, family, and work relationships. It's also possible that they're looking for specific information, like which treatments and doctors are the best. In personal communications from people who belong to online Behçet's support groups, one of the top reasons given for **not** posting to their group(s) is the feeling that their own symptoms are too mild. They don't want to complain when other patients seem to have it worse.

82. What are the chances I'll be hospitalized at some point with Behçet's complications?

The only study about hospitalization of Behçet's patients was done in 2013.[5] It looked at the medical records of people seen in a Behçet's clinic in Turkey over 10 years. Only 178 of the 4,000 treated patients (4%) had to be hospitalized, and they were admitted a total of 211 times. Three-quarters of these patients were men. Table 14.1 gives a breakdown of the reasons for admission.

Table 14.1 Reasons for 211 hospitalizations of 178 Behçet's patients over 10 years in a Turkish clinic (2002–2011)

Reason for hospitalization	Number of hospitalizations	% of total hospitalizations
Behçet's organ involvement	118 out of 211	56%
Vascular involvement [a]	74 out of 118	63%

Reason for hospitalization	Number of hospitalizations	% of total hospitalizations
Neurologic involvement [b]	14	12%
GI involvement	6	5%
Eye involvement (uveitis)	6	5%
Complications	93 out of 211	44%
Infections	39 out of 93	42%
Drug-related problems (adverse events) [c]	15	16%
Cancer [d]	4	4%
Unspecified	42	38%

[a] = 21 patients with pulmonary artery aneurysms, 10 with peripheral artery aneurysms and 11 with venous thrombosis (e.g., superior vena cava thrombosis and Budd–Chiari syndrome)
[b] = 10 patients with parenchymal involvement (brain, brainstem or spinal cord inflammation); 1 had dural sinus thrombosis (blood clot in vessels leading from the brain); 2 unspecified
[c] = Unspecified problems with azathioprine, cyclophosphamide and infliximab
[d] = Acute myeloblastic leukemia, non-Hodgkin's lymphoma, mesothelioma, unknown adenocarcinoma. Unclear if these cancers were directly related to Behçet's.

You can see that the number of hospitalizations in this report was small—only 4% of all patients seen in the clinic were admitted— and most of them were male. Since more American women than men have Behçet's, it would be interesting to see results from a hospitalization study done with US patients.

83. What's the life expectancy for someone with Behçet's?

This number may vary depending on your location, but many Behçet's patients live as long as "regular" (healthy) people. In a group of five studies that included more than 4,700 BD patients (with over 4,200 of those patients in Japan and Korea, 316 patients in Morocco, and 152 in Turkey),[6] death rates from Behçet's-related symptoms or complications ranged from 0% to about 4%. In other words, out of any group of 100 people with BD, up to four people in the group might die of BD-related issues over time. A 2014 French study found very different mortality rates, though, between BD patients they'd followed for 15 years from Europe, North African countries (Morocco, Algeria, Tunisia, and Egypt) and sub-Saharan Africa (the remaining 51 countries in Africa). There was a 6% mortality rate in European patients after 15 years, a 9% rate for North African patients, and a much higher 19% rate for those in sub-Saharan Africa.[7] A 2003 Turkish study found that 10% of their patients who were followed over 20 years eventually died of BD-related symptoms or complications.[2] More studies are needed, because mortality rates seem to differ widely based on the country and/or available treatment options.

No matter which studies and statistics you look at, though, two groups of BD patients are most at risk: young males between the ages of 14–24, followed by young males from 25–34. Involvement of blood vessels (like aneurysms and clots) and/or the central nervous system add to the risks. Possible life-threatening problems, if they're going to happen, occur most often during the first seven years after BD symptoms start. The threat goes down steadily after that. It's the opposite of diseases like lupus and rheumatoid arthritis,[6] where the risk of death for patients goes *up* as they age. The BD patients that are least at risk are women of any age, and men from 35–50.

What are the Behçet's-related issues to watch out for? Table 14.2 gives a breakdown.

Table 14.2 Causes of death in 42 of 387 Behçet's patients followed for 20 years in Turkey [2]

Reason for death	Number of patients	%
Large-vessel disease[a]	17 of 42 patients	41%
Central nervous system involvement[b]	5	12%
Heart disease[c]	5	12%
Kidney disease[d]	4	10%
Cancer[e]	4	10%
Other [f]	4	10%
Unknown	3	7%

[a] = Pulmonary artery aneurysm (PAA) in 9; Budd-Chiari syndrome in 3; vena cava occlusion in 4; abdominal aorta aneurysm in 1
[b] = Severe, recurrent, progressive CNS parenchymal disease in 5 (inflammation in or around the brain, brainstem or spinal cord)
[c] = Congestive heart failure in 2; coronary artery disease in 3
[d] = Kidney failure from amyloidosis in 2; chronic kidney failure in 2
[e] = Non-Hodgkin's lymphoma in 1; lung cancer in 1; gastric cancer in 1; kidney cancer in 1
[f] = Stroke in 1; suicide in 2; traffic accident in 1

After reading this section, you may be worrying even more about your own (or your loved one's) future. Don't. If you've read through the rest of this book, you already know the basics: No one has figured out the cause of Behçet's, and there seem to be big differences in the level of symptoms and outcomes from country to country.

If you live in the United States or Western Europe, very little research has been done on Behçet's in those areas compared to Silk Road countries. As a result, we still don't know how much of the Middle- and Far-Eastern research actually applies to the West. If you've met other people with BD through online groups, you've probably already grasped how different we all are. For example, drugs that work well for one person may not work at all for others. The best advice? Try to stay optimistic. Treatments are *much* more effective now than the ones available 30+ years ago, and it's expected that this positive trend—and research—will continue.

References

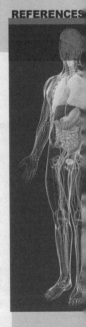

REFERENCES

CHAPTER 14

1. 2012 Annual Statistical Report on the Social Security Disability Insurance Program (released November 2013). Available at http://www.ssa.gov/policy/docs/statcomps/di_asr/2012/index.html

2. Kural-Seyahi, E., Fresko, I., Seyahi, N., Ozyazgan, Y., Mat, C., Hamuryudan, V., Yurdakul, S., & Yazici, H. (2003). The long-term mortality and morbidity of Behçet's syndrome: a 2-decade outcome survey of 387 patients followed at a dedicated center. *Medicine (Baltimore), 82(1),* 60–76.

3. Sibley, C., Yazici, Y., Tascilar, K., Khan, N., Bata, Y., Yazici, H., Goldbach-Mansky, R., & Hatemi, G. (2014). Behçet Syndrome Manifestations and Activity in the United States versus Turkey - A Cross-sectional Cohort Comparison. *The Journal of rheumatology. Advance online publication.* pii: jrheum.131227.

4. Davis, G. L. & Brissett, D. (1993). Experiencing Behçet's Disease: A View From 245 Patients. In B. Wechsler & P. Godeau (Eds.), *Behçet's Disease* (pp. 211-214). Amsterdam: Excerpta Medica.

5. Ozguler, Y., Pala, A. S., Hamuryudan V., Hatemi, G., Yurdakul, S., & Yazici, H. (2013). Causes of hospitalisation in Behçet's syndrome over a ten-year period. *Annals of the Rheumatic Diseases, 72*(Suppl 3), 936. (Presentation at 2013 EULAR Congress).

6. Seyahi, E., & Yazici, H. (2010). Prognosis in Behçet's syndrome. In Yazici, H. & Yazici, Y. (Eds.), *Behçet's Syndrome* (pp. 285-298). New York, NY: Springer.

7. Savey, L., Resche-Rigon, M., Wechsler, B., Comarmond, C., Piette, J. C., Cacoub, P., & Saadoun, D. (2014). Ethnicity and association with disease manifestations and mortality in Behçet's disease. *Orphanet journal of rare diseases, 9*(42). Available online at http://www.ojrd.com/content/pdf/1750-1172-9-42.pdf.

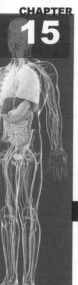

CHAPTER 15

Miscellaneous questions: Sleep, vitamin D, tattoos, sex, teeth, fibromyalgia and joints, flu shots, and genitourinary issues

84. Can Behçet's cause sleep problems?

Yes. One out of every four people with BD actually sleeps less than five hours every night.[1] This sleep deficit can happen even when BDers aren't taking prednisone or other medications known to disturb sleep.

Restless legs syndrome (RLS) tops the list of sleep disorders in BD patients. RLS causes creeping or crawling feelings at rest, usually in the lower legs. Moving the legs helps relieve the sensation. RLS gets more common in people with BD as they age.[2]

Learn more about restless legs syndrome in the NIH information booklet on the CD that accompanies this book.

ON THE CD

Obstructive sleep apnea (OSA) is second on the list of sleep disorders for BD patients after restless legs syndrome. Like RLS, it's much more common in people with Behçet's than it is in the general population. OSA causes a person who's asleep to temporarily stop breathing and wake up, often many times per hour.[1]

As you might expect, a BD patient with either of these problems may feel more tired and sleepy than normal during the day. Research shows that if fibromyalgia is added to the mix, a Behçet's patient's daytime fatigue could reach a severe level. This situation can be compounded by the serious fatigue and pain already felt by many people with autoimmune/rheumatic diseases.[3]

Finally, narcolepsy is a problem for a small number of people with Behçet's; it causes a person to fall asleep suddenly, even in the middle of an activity. Narcolepsy includes a few other issues besides these sudden-sleep episodes, such as sleep paralysis (where you're temporarily unable to move or speak when waking up or going to sleep), hypnagogic and hynopompic hallucinations (vividly seeing or hearing things that aren't there while you're on the verge of falling asleep or waking up), and cataplexy (where sudden muscle weakness happens in part or all of your body, often caused by strong emotions like fear).[4]

85. Do Behçet's patients have low levels of vitamin D?

That seems to be the case, but some researchers may not have looked at all of the reasons for their BD patients' vitamin D levels. For example, vitamin D levels may be affected by obesity; smoking; the aging process; low estrogen levels; other autoimmune diseases like lupus and MS; and the use of many different drugs. Some of these drugs include blood thinners; anti-seizure meds; some blood pressure medications; water pills (diuretics); weight-loss drugs like Xenical; cholesterol-lowering drugs like Questran; and prednisone and other steroids. Colchicine may also affect vitamin D levels in some people. Read the two articles on Behçet's and vitamin D that are listed in the References section at the end of the chapter,[5,6] and speak with your doctor for more information.

About one out of every three people diagnosed with Behçet's develops a problem with their health and/or their tattoo(s) as a result of the tattoo process.[7] In comparison, only one out of every 10 supposedly-healthy people reports a post-tattoo problem.[8] Problems may include pain, some swelling, fluid discharge, minor bleeding, redness, tenderness, crusting, itching, and/or a skin rash. According to personal communication with a 12-year veteran tattoo artist who also has Behçet's, tattoo healing issues aren't just common to BD patients, though: people who are diabetic, anemic, take certain medications like blood thinners or immunosuppressants, or have other autoimmune disorders may also experience healing problems.[22] It's possible that Behçet's could make some of these tattoo complications worse; in a way, it's a variation on the pathergy response (see Question 11).

This author sent an informal survey about tattoo experiences to three online Behçet's support groups in 2014; 73 BD patients with tattoos responded.[7] About one out of every three Behçet's patients (29%) who'd gotten tattoos before they were diagnosed—and before they'd had any Behçet's-type symptoms—said they'd had issues with their tattoos while they healed. Slightly more, though, (34%), had problems if they'd gotten their tattoos *after* being diagnosed with Behçet's.

Getting tattooed before <u>and</u> after a BD diagnosis

Twenty-six of the 73 patients in the Behçet's tattoo survey got tattoos both before they were diagnosed with Behçet's (or started showing BD-type symptoms) **and** after they were diagnosed. Types of "tattoo problems" referred to in Figure 15.1 include excessive swelling of the tattooed area; a pathergy-type reaction (pustules—like whiteheads—on parts of the tattoo); infection; "angry" skin rashes; a new flare of BD symptoms within 1-7 days of getting tattooed (after being diagnosed with Behçet's); an unusually long healing time; and a strong reaction to one or more ink colors.

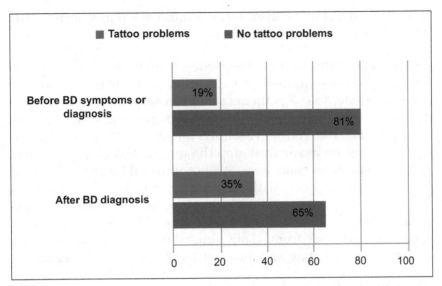

Tattoo problems   **No tattoo problems**

Before BD symptoms or diagnosis: 19% / 81%

After BD diagnosis: 35% / 65%

▲ Figure 15.1
Results of tattoo sessions on 26 BD patients who were tattooed before **and** after their Behçet's diagnosis or start of BD-type symptoms
Source: J. Zeis, 2014

A sampling of comments from tattooed BD patients includes the following: "Would not hold color and had to have it recolored twice; did not have this problem with black ink"; "When the pustules from the pathergy response [on my ankle tattoo] opened or burst, they would [also] leak clear fluid or ink. Now the tattoo is very faded and uneven and almost entirely gone in small, patchy spots"; "Got a cyst"; "The tattoo is still sensitive to the touch almost two years later"; "Some colors didn't take or stick. Formed thick scabs around some of the outlines"; "Had to go back after it healed because the bright pink ink wouldn't stay. He kept trying to color it [but still] in some parts there is little or no color. He said he hadn't seen anything like this before"; "Part of it kept coming off like my body was rejecting the ink"; and "I was diagnosed nine years after getting the tattoo, and five years into having Behçet's, my tattoo would randomly bubble up and become three-dimensional. This would only happen to the tattoo; no ulcers anywhere, no Behçet's symptoms." [After the survey ended, seven additional BD patients contacted the author with the same type of inflamed "3D tattoo" experience; this problem recurs for them at random, even years after being tattooed.] Several people also mentioned problems with excessive bleeding during the tattoo procedure, although one person with that issue actually had a clotting disorder. It's unknown if any of these BD patients were taking blood thinners at the time.

Some people who **don't** have Behçet's have developed uveitis and the above-mentioned "3D elevation" of their new tattoos at the same time, too.[9] Erythema nodosum has also been reported after tattooing, along with individual reports of other serious eye problems, like retinal vasculitis and cystoid macular edema. Oral prednisone has helped stop the uveitis and skin flares, but they've sometimes come back; it's not unusual for these tattoo(s) to swell again, timed with another uveitis flare-up. There is one report of three people with this type of recurring eye/tattoo inflammation who took the extreme step of having their tattoos removed (cut out) from their skin. Afterwards, their uveitis cleared up completely and no other treatments were needed.[9]

What do doctors and tattoo artists suggest for any people with chronic illness who want to get a tattoo?

- Speak with your doctor **before** getting a tattoo, especially if you've had pathergy-type reactions in the past or problems with healing, or if you're taking any of the following medications: aspirin or other blood thinners; anti-TNF drugs or immunosuppressants (including prednisone); or Accutane or other meds that can cause skin sensitivity. (This list is not complete, so ask your healthcare provider.)
- Get your tattoo at a licensed, professional studio that's clean and where equipment is disinfected between customers.
- Make sure the tattoo artist wears gloves and changes them between clients.
- Tell the tattoo artist in advance about any medications you're taking, and follow his or her care instructions as your tattoo heals.
- If you have any autoimmune condition, including BD, make sure you're not flaring or sick when you get your tattoo, and keep your tattoo sessions short. Women who normally flare around their periods may want to wait until after menstruation before getting tattooed.
- It's rare but still possible for tattoos to cause endocarditis (inflammation of the inside lining of the heart) or systemic vasculitis within the first two weeks of healing.

If you have a fever that won't go away, or joint pains and/or muscle aches after getting a tattoo, see your doctor to check for an infection or other health issue.[8]

87. Can Behçet's cause sexual problems?

Yes, but it may take some time to sort out the specific reasons for it. Sexual problems in a person with Behçet's can have a physical cause, an emotional cause, or both. Problems can include issues like frequency of sex, ability to talk about your sexual needs, level of sexual satisfaction, active avoidance of sex, touching, painful intercourse, inability to have an orgasm, inability to get or keep an erection, and premature ejaculation. Some of these sexual problems could be directly caused by Behçet's-related nerve or blood-vessel damage, or by things like medications, alcohol or substance use, menopause, hormone levels, aging, emotional issues like depression, or by other illnesses like diabetes.

A 2013 study of sexual function in BD patients with or without depression[10] came up with these results:

- Almost all of the Behçet's patients who were depressed had sexual problems. BD patients who weren't depressed did a little better: only three out of every five of these patients had sexual problems.
- Significantly more women with Behçet's than healthy women have issues with sexual satisfaction, avoidance of sex, painful intercourse, and an inability to have an orgasm.
- Significantly more men with Behçet's than healthy men have issues with impotence, premature ejaculation, sexual satisfaction, and frequency of sex.
- Genital ulcers can play a big part in BD patients' levels of sexual satisfaction, their avoidance of sex, painful intercourse, and inability to have an orgasm.

88. Can dental problems be related to Behçet's?

Yes. Here are results from a few different research studies:[11,12,13]

- About three out of every five Behçet's patients (60%) have a history of frequent tonsillitis and many cavities ("decay, mottling, and fillings" in 15 or more teeth) before any of their BD symptoms start.

- Once their Behçet's-related symptoms begin, most of these patients keep having problems with tonsillitis and cavities. Compared to healthy people of the same age, they need to have more dental treatments and more of their teeth pulled.
- Due to the pain of mouth ulcers, many Behçet's patients don't brush their teeth regularly or floss. As a result, their gums may be more inflamed, and they may have more plaque buildup than healthy people.
- BD patients who have more gum disease, deep pockets (areas where the gums have pulled away from the teeth), and plaque buildup may develop a more severe case of Behçet's.
- Even though dental cleanings and treatments may cause flares in the short term, Behçet's patients may have *fewer* mouth ulcers and other BD symptoms long-term if they see the dentist every six months and get regular cleanings to eliminate any infections.
- Besides having symptom flares after dental treatments and cleanings, many BD patients also report symptom flares after tooth extractions and after episodes of tonsillitis.
- An uncommon type of *Streptococcus sanguis* has been found in the mouths of up to 70% of BD patients, although it's still not proven to be a cause of Behçet's. Many personal BD contacts, though, report a long history of strep throat infections before developing their first Behçet's-related symptoms.

89. Do Behçet's patients have a problem with fibromyalgia?

Yes, some do. If you put 100 people with BD in a room, anywhere from six to 37 of them could have fibromyalgia. Most of the affected people will be women.[14,15]

ON THE CD

Go to the CD to read the NIH information booklet on fibromyalgia.

A diagnosis of fibromyalgia is based on the American College of Rheumatology's (ACR) guidelines: a person must have a history of widespread pain for at least three months and have at least 11 of the 18 tender points shown in Figure 15.2. "Widespread pain" means pain in four different areas of the body at the same time:

on the left and right sides of the body, and above and below the waist. Other health issues that can show up in BD patients with fibromyalgia include fatigue, morning tiredness, stiffness, and anxiety.[14]

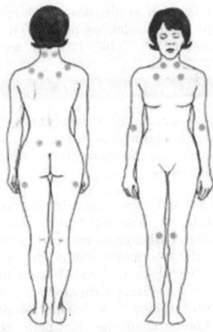

▲ Figure 15.2
Location of nine paired tender points in the American College of Rheumatology criteria for fibromyalgia
Source: http://www.niams.nih.gov/Health_Info/Fibromyalgia/

90. What types of joint involvement are common?[16,17]

Arthritis and arthralgia (joint pain) are common in Behçet's. For example, about half of all BD patients in the United States have some type of joint involvement. Joint pain and inflammation often comes and goes, with each episode lasting from days to weeks. Joint pain is also "migratory" in some cases: it may move unexpectedly from one part of the body to joints in other areas.

Most people with BD-related joint pain are affected in the larger joints of the body, like the knees, wrists, ankles, and elbows, although the hands and/or feet can be involved, too. Pain may be in just one joint or in several at the same time. This type of inflammation is called "non-erosive" because it hardly ever destroys the joints. In rare situations, though, a Behçet's patient may have destruction in the joints that looks like a case of rheumatoid arthritis or psoriatic arthritis instead.

Like many BD symptoms, joint pain may be hard to treat. Trial-and-error may be needed to find the best drug or combination of drugs for each patient. NSAIDs such as piroxicam (Feldene), anti-TNF drugs like infliximab (Remicade), or pentoxifylline (Trental) may help. See Question 73, Table 13.1 for more treatment options.

91. Is it safe to get flu shots if you have Behçet's?[18]

Yes, as long as the flu shot doesn't contain live viruses, it doesn't include an *adjuvant* (a substance sometimes added to vaccines to increase your immune response), and there's no other medical reason why you shouldn't be vaccinated.

When researchers vaccinated some Behçet's patients against the H1N1 flu virus, they found the flu shots didn't work as well for people who were having a lot of BD symptoms at the time of the injection. Taking typical BD treatments like prednisone, immunosuppressants, or anti-TNF drugs had no effect on the shot's level of protection. In general, Behçet's patients had more temporary side effects with the flu shot than healthy people did. These side effects included fever, headache, joint pain, and muscle pain. More research is being done to find out if a second vaccination during flu season would provide a higher level of protection for BD patients.

92. What are some genitourinary problems linked to Behçet's?[19,20,21]

• While these issues are rare in some countries, men and boys with Behçet's may still develop **orchitis** (inflammation of the testicle), **epididymitis** (inflammation of the coiled tube at the back of the testicle that collects and transfers sperm), or **varicocele** (swelling of the veins in the scrotum). Orchitis and epididymitis may cause fever along with sudden pain and swelling in one or both testicles.

Read more information about getting flu vaccinations when you have Behçet's:

ON THE WEB

http://behcets.blogspot.com/2010/09/getting-flu-vaccinations-when-youhave.html

- It's possible to have repeated bouts of **urethritis** (inflammation of the urethra) and/or sterile **cystitis** (a bladder infection or a UTI: urinary tract infection) when you have BD. Lesions/ulcers may also be found in the **urethra** and **bladder**.
- Other types of kidney involvement in Behçet's are uncommon, but may include **hematuria** (blood in the urine); **proteinuria** (protein in the urine); **AA type amyloidosis** (deposits of a protein called amyloid in the kidneys, liver or spleen, which it may lead to kidney failure); and **glomerulonephritis** (inflammation of glomeruli in the kidneys, which are small blood vessels that help filter your blood and get rid of extra fluid).

References

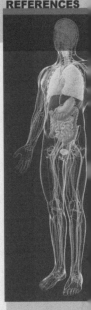

CHAPTER 15

1. Tascilar, N. F., Tekin, N. S., Ankarali, H., Sezer, T., Atik, L., Emre, U., Duysak, S., & Cinar, F. (2011). Sleep disorders in Behçet's disease, and their relationship with fatigue and quality of life. *Journal of sleep research, 21(3)*, 281–288. Available online at http://onlinelibrary.wiley.com/doi/10.1111/j.1365-2869.2011.00976.x/pdf

2. Ediz, L., Hiz, O., Toprak, M., Ceylan, M. F., Yazmalar, L., & Gulcu, E. (2011). Restless legs syndrome in Behçet's disease. *The Journal of international medical research, 39(3)*, 759–765.

3. Geenen, R., Overman, C. L., Da Silva, J. A. P., & Kool, M. B. (2014). Severe fatigue is highly prevalent in all rheumatic diseases: An international study. *Annals of the rheumatic diseases, 73*(Suppl 2), doi:10.1136/annrheumdis-2014-eular.2399. Available online at http://www.abstracts2view.com/eular/view.php?nu=EULAR14L_THU0593-HPR

4. Hsieh, C. F., Lai, C. L., Liu, C. K., Lan, S. H., Hsieh, S. W., & Hsu, C. Y. (2009). Narcolepsy and Behcet's disease: report of a Chinese-Taiwanese case. *Sleep medicine, 11(4)*, 427–428.

5. Karatay, S., Yildirim, K., Karakuzu, A., Kiziltunc, A., Engin, R. I., Eren, Y. B., & Aktas, A. (2011). Vitamin D status in patients with Behcet's Disease. *Clinics (Sao Paulo, Brazil), 66(5)*, 721–723. Available online at http://www.ncbi.nlm.nih.gov/pmc/articles/PMC3109365/pdf/cln-66-05-721.pdf

6. Ganeb, S. S., Sabry, H. H., El-Assal, M. M., Kamal, H. M., & Fayed, A. A. (2013). Vitamin D levels in patients with Behcet's disease: Significance and impact on disease measures. *The Egyptian Rheumatologist, 35*(3), 151-157. Available online at http://www.sciencedirect.com/science/article/pii/S1110116413000173

7. Zeis, J. (2014). Preliminary results of informal tattoo survey in three online Behçet's support groups. Unpublished.

8. Kluger, N. (2012). Acute complications of tattooing presenting in the ED. *The American journal of emergency medicine, 30(9)*, 2055–2063.

9. Ostheimer, T. A., Burkholder, B. M., Leung, T. G., Butler, N. J., Dunn, J. P., & Thorne, J. E. (2014). Tattoo-Associated Uveitis. *American journal of ophthalmology*, doi:10.1016/j.ajo.2014.05.019.

10. Gul, I. G., Kartalci, S., Cumurcu, B. E., Karincaoglu,Y., Yologlu, S., & Karlidag, R. (2012). Evaluation of sexual function in patients presenting with Behçet's disease with or without depression. *Journal of the European Academy of Dermatology and Venereology : JEADV, 27(10)*, 1244–1251.

11. Tsuchida, M., Mineshita, S., Okonogi, H., Sugimori, K., Hoshi, K., Horiuchi, T., Wang, L. M., & Fujimoto, E. K. (1997). The role of an uncommon type of oral streptococcus sanguis in the etiology of behcet's disease. *Environmental health and preventive medicine, 2(2)*, 59–63. Available online at http://www.ncbi.nlm.nih.gov/pmc/articles/PMC2723434/

12. Mumcu, G. (2008). Behçet's disease: a dentist's overview. *Clinical and experimental rheumatology, 26(4 Suppl 50)*, S121-4. Available online at http://www.clinexprheumatol.org/article.asp?a=3453

13. Mumcu, G., Ergun, T., Inanc, N., Fresko, I., Atalay, T., Hayran, O., & Direskeneli, H. (2004). Oral health is impaired in Behçet's disease and is associated with disease severity. *Rheumatology (Oxford, England), 43(8)*, 1028–1033. Available online at http://rheumatology.oxfordjournals.org/content/43/8/1028.long

14. Lee, S. S., Yoon, H. J., Chang, H. K., & Park, K. S. (2005). Fibromyalgia in Behçet's disease is associated with anxiety and depression, and not with disease activity. *Clinical and experimental rheumatology, 23 (Suppl 38)*, S15-9. Available online at http://www.clinexprheumatol.org/article.asp?a=2718

15. Haliloglu, S., Carlioglu, A., Akdeniz, D., Karaaslan, Y., & Kosar, A. (2014). Fibromyalgia in patients with other rheumatic diseases: prevalence and relationship with disease activity. *Rheumatology international, doi:10.1007/s00296-014-2972-8.*

16. Bicer, A. (2012). Musculoskeletal Findings in Behcet's Disease. *Pathology research international*, doi:10.1155/2012/653806. *Available online at* http://www.ncbi.nlm.nih.gov/pmc/articles/PMC3180072/

17. Yurdakul, S., Yazici, H., Tuzun, Y., Pazarli, H., Yalcin, B., Altac, M., Ozyazgan, Y., Tuzuner, N., & Muftuoglu, A. (1983). The arthritis of Behçet's disease: a prospective study. *Annals of the rheumatic diseases, 42(5)*, 505–515. Available online at http://ard.bmj.com/content/42/5/505.long

18. Prado, L. L., Saad, C. G. S., Moraes, J. C. B., Ribeiro, A. C. M., Aikawa, N. E., Silva, C. A., Schainberg, C. G...& Goncalves, C. (2013) Behçet's Disease Activity: An Important Factor For Immunogenicity Of Unadjuvanted Influenza A/H1N1 Vaccine. *Arthritis & Rheumatism, 65*(10 Supp), S744. Available online at https://ww2.rheumatology.org/apps/MyAnnualMeeting/Abstract/36846

19. Calamia, K. T. & Fresko, I. (2010). Miscellaneous manifestations of Behçet's Disease. In Yazici, H. & Yazici, Y. (Eds.), *Behçet's Syndrome.* (pp. 193-200). New York, NY: Springer.

20. Plotkin, G. R. (1988). Miscellaneous clinical manifestations, Part II. In Plotkin, G. R., Calabro, J. J. & O'Duffy, J. D. (Eds.). *Behçet's Disease: A Contemporary Synopsis.* (pp. 256-257). Mount Kisco, NY: Futura Publishing.

21. Korkmaz, C., Ozcan, A., & Akcar, N. (2005). Increased frequency of ultrasonographic findings suggestive of renal stones in patients with ankylosing spondylitis. *Clinical and experimental rheumatology, 23(3)*, 389–392. Available online at http://www.clinexprheumatol.org/article.asp?a=2606

22. S. Zrinko, Inksanity Tattoos (personal communication, August 11, 2014).

About the CD-ROM

The CD-ROM that accompanies this book includes the following files and information:

- **NIHinfo:** 95 booklets and handouts from the NIH that deal with a variety of medical information related to Behcet's disease.
- **BDmap:** A map showing the worldwide distribution of Behcet's disease as of 2014.
- **CircSys:** An illustration showing all veins and arteries of the circulatory system.
- **Docs&Gp:** This PDF includes lists and links of:
  - o   International specialists and treatment centers
  - o   International Behcet's organizations
  - o   International Behcet's online support groups
  - o   Miscellaneous resources administered by Joanne Zeis
  - o   Other books by Joanne Zeis

- **NoDiag:** Tips for undiagnosed people, from the NIH Office of Rare Diseases Research.
- **OnWebLk**: A listing of all "On the Web" links from each chapter in the book.
- **PAFinfo**: Helpful information and links from the Patient Advocate Foundation.
- **Refs**: Links to all journal abstracts and articles that are listed in the references at the end of each chapter.
- **Videos**: Links to an assortment of videos about Behcet's disease and vasculitis.

Index

A

ABDA (the American Behçet's Disease Association), 3
Abnormal lab and blood test results in Behçet's patients, 14
American College of Rheumatology's (ACR), 116
ASCA (Antisaccharomyces Cerevisiae Antibodies), 54

B

Behcet's disease (BD), 1
  common symptoms of, 9
  common types of joint involvement in, 117
  dental problems and, 115
  diagnosis of, 14
  differences between patients in different countries (table), 11
  fibromyalgia and, 116
  genitourinary problems and, 118
    orchitis, 118
    epididymitis, 118
    varicocele, 118
    urethritis, 120
    hematuria, 120
    proteinuria, 120
    amyloidosis, 120
    glomerulonephritis, 120
  link with the old "Silk Road" trade routes, 6, 10
  other names of, 2
  prevalence rates of (table), 7–8
  safety to use flu shots, 118
  sex problems and, 115
  signs, symptoms and prognosis of, 13
  sleep problems and BD, 110
    restless legs syndrome (RLS), 110
    obstructive sleep apnea (OSA), 111
  symptoms of, 1
  tattooing problems for BS patients, 113
    doctors and tattoo artists suggest, 114
    getting tattooed before and after a BD diagnosis, 112
  vitamin D levels and BD patients, 111
Behçet's Disease Current Activity Form (BDCAF), 20
Behcet genetic, 76
  children and, 76
  family members and, 77
  features of, 76
  genetic anticipation, 78
  neonatal BD, 87
  symptoms of BD in children, 78, 79
Behçet's syndrome, 2
Behçet's Syndrome Center, 3
Behçet's Syndrome Centres of Excellence, 3
Benign paroxysmal positional vertigo (BPPV), 60
Budd-Chiari syndrome (BCS), 69

C

Caloric stimulation test, 61
Cardiovascular system and BD, 64
  artery-related problems for BD patients, 69
  blood vessel problems and BD, 67
  heart problems and BD patients (table), 64
  symptoms pointing to heart involvement, 66
  vein-related problems for BD patients, 68
Crampy pain, 55
Cerebrospinal fluid (CSF) analysis, 40
CVST (cerebral venous sinus thrombosis), 78
Claudication, 68

D

Deep vein thrombosis (DVT), 10, 68, 73, 86